Fire Your Doctor
Cure Yourself

PAUL KEENAN

Copyright Notice

Email: paulkeenan@antarana.com

Web address: http://www.antarana.com/books.html

FIND ME ON FACEBOOK

https://www.facebook.com/PaulKeenanAuthor/

Important Notice

"You know you suffered many years with physical and psychological disorders?" prodded the Naturopath I interviewed only a few days ago.

"Yes", I responded.

"And you know you travelled the world looking for cures?"

"Uh-huh", I replied, wondering where this was heading.

"I could have cured you in three days".

Foreword

What do you do in an Age where physical and mental disorders are spiralling out of control and Doctors cannot or will not cure? When over-the-counter products are a waste of money and Alternatives cannot cure either? When you are overwhelmed with information from experts, none of whom agree with each other, and complicated medical jargon leaves you totally confused and paralyzed with indecision?

When years of modern medicine proved ineffective and harmful, in resolving his own physical and mental disorders, Paul Keenan turned to Alternatives. Over two decades there was hardly a therapy he did not try. Frustrated by the inability of both modern and alternative medicine to cure him and close to breakdown, Paul was left with no choice. He FIRED HIS DOCTORS, fleeing abroad, in a desperate attempt to save his sanity and recover his health. When, in an Indian backwater, a traditional Ayurvedic healer reversed his arthritis, Paul's eyes were opened to the power of Natural Healing. Inspired by his experience, Paul spent the following years, studying and experimenting with the methods of the great healing masters, to better understand what makes us sick and what is needed, to get well.

Finding time between running Wellness Retreats and online Health Coaching, Paul brings us 'Fire Your Doctor Cure Yourself'. Presenting, in plain language, the latest research, forgotten ancient knowledge, a dose of common sense and simple, proven methods of healing, to offer new hope.

Dedication

This book is dedicated to my dear mother, who did not deserve to suffer as she did. If she were still here, I would wrap her in my arms and apologize for my lack of understanding of just how sick she was. Instead, I have written this book to honour her memory and the memory of untold millions like her who, desperately needing cures, died disappointed

I also dedicate this book to my children, Michael, Lauren and Neil, who wanted their father to be a hero, only to find he was mortal

Finally, I dedicate this book to YOU. The courageous person seeking to reverse your disease who knows, instinctively, nature holds the key

Acknowledgments

I would like to acknowledge the champions of the last century, who fought to bring important healing knowledge to the world.

Dr John Christopher, Dr Max Gerson and his daughter Charlotte, Dr Richard Schulze, Linus Pauling, Dr Abram Hoffer, Gandhi, who established 'Nature Cure' Centres throughout India, and the traditional Ayurvedic healers I met, who with compassion, devotion and skill, showed me a better way.

I would also like to thank Dr Paul Johnson for his awesome intellect, uncritical support and for being so generous with his time.

Who Should Buy This Book?

Everyone! At the rates of sickness we see in the West, you are virtually guaranteed to experience one or more chronic, degenerative disorders by the time you are 50.

Cancer

Heart Disease

Diabetes and Prediabetes

Arthritis

Obesity

Anxiety, Depression, Bipolar, ADHD, Addiction

Fibromyalgia

Hypertension

Allergies

Alzheimer's, Parkinson's and Dementia

Asthma

Chronic Fatigue Syndrome

AIDS

Gastrointestinal Diseases - Crohn's, Colitis, Celiac, Diverticulitis, IBS

Metabolic Disorder

Autoimmune Disorders – including MS and Rheumatoid Arthritis

Many others!

"Guests arrive with a cloud over their heads and leave with a spring in their step. It's a remarkable transformation"

Paul Keenan

TABLE OF CONTENTS

Dan

84 year old Canadian, Dan, was a gentle giant. When he came shuffling up my drive, he couldn't bend his fingers, they were so swollen with Rheumatoid Arthritis. Dan was 40kg overweight and down in the dumps. A big meat-eater all his life, he told me about his triple heart-bypass, his Cancer and how the medications he was taking only made his Arthritis worse. Dan had certainly experienced his share of illness. I am too old", he said. "The Doctors have written me off".

Alternative practitioners refused to help Dan because he was high risk. They do not have the protection of the State and could go to jail if Dan suddenly dropped dead on their doorstep. I explained, for the same reason, I could not help.

"Please", said Dan. "Nobody else will help me".

My heart went out to this dignified man so I recommended a simple program with a long track record of success and safety. Dan came off most of his medications and commenced a citrus-based, juice fast. Like most people Dan could not imagine going two hours without eating but nevertheless committed to the program. After 7 days Dan was feeling so well he asked if he could do 3 more. After 10 he called again and said he was feeling even better and could he do 14? I suggested he stop at 14. On the morning of the 15th day, Dan walked up my drive, transformed. He had lost 9kgs, looked ten years younger, his Arthritis symptoms were gone and his depression had lifted. It was wonderful to see.

"How did you get on with the juices?" I asked.

"It was easy after the first day", said Dan. "I wish I could have continued".

Introduction

"You're FIRED!"

More of us should try it, don't you think? Walk into our Doctor's office, look them in the eye and give it to them straight. If you think about it, the idea you would buy a book titled 'Fire Your Doctor Cure Yourself' is an act of independence and defiance some might consider revolutionary. I am sure you were not thinking that when you picked this off the bookshelf or ordered it online. You just want to know how to fix your Arthritis or Cancer or Diabetes or Allergies.

Welcome to the 'Bypass Age'. An Age where, if Doctors cannot or will not cure, you bypass them. An Age where, if drug corporations, Medical Associations, 'captured' Consumer Protection Agencies and 'revolving-door', government flunkies erect barriers to change, you bypass them, too. Around 50% of patients are now using CAM (Complementary and Alternative Medicine), bypassing their Doctors.

A revolution in Health Care is occurring and is certainly needed. We are the sickest species on the planet and getting sicker. Mankind cannot sustain this expensive, technological-chemical assault on our bodies, minds and environment, for much longer. The number of us succumbing to chronic, degenerative disorders is too great. Perhaps it will come when half of our children are Autistic (as projected). Perhaps it will come when more than half of us die from Cancer (we are almost there now). When corporations make more money curing disease than treating it. Or, as a Doctor friend bluntly put it,

"When the owners and CEOs of 'Big Food', 'Big Pharma' and the vaccine makers are all swinging from the same branch."

It is coming. I hear it with every phone call and from every visitor I receive. They may use different words but the message is the same:

"I am sick and my Doctor cannot cure me."

An explosion of interest in Natural and Alternative methods of healing is happening and you and I are part of it. Quite when we reach the point where wholesale change will come is hard to say. It isn't just Health Care which needs to change. Doctors are those we see AFTER we have fallen ill. What is making us sick BEFORE we see the Doctor also needs to change. The choices you and I make, every single day, consciously or unconsciously, which build health or build disease. Think about that. Every choice you make is either building health or building disease. Are you aware of this? Or is your health "The Doctor's job"?

You may not realize it but you are part of a massive shift in human awareness. For the first time in the history of mankind we have access to knowledge the rich and powerful traditionally held. Instant access to more information, in one hour on the internet, than we had in a lifetime, 100 years ago. It is a wonderful window of opportunity which, unfortunately, is closing, with our every keystroke and mouse movement tracked and archived and internet giants increasing their filtering of what we are allowed to see. When my mother died a painful and undignified death there was no internet and no hope. You accepted what Doctors told you, without question, because 'The Doctor knows best'. Now we understand this is not true. Doctors know only what they have been taught. They treat, only in a way they are allowed to treat. They know nothing about alternatives, ignore patients' individual differences, pay lip-service to prevention, and their grandmothers know more about nutrition than they do. Today, thanks to the internet, within minutes of your Doctor declaring your condition 'incurable', putting you on a lifetime regime of colourful pills (while cruelly extinguishing hope anything else can cure you), you can be online, discovering simple, safe healing methods you never knew existed. Whether they work or not I will come to but at least you know of their existence.

When I first started researching Rheumatoid Arthritis (RA), the disease that killed my mother, my knowledge of medicine and the health system was non-existent. I was strong (apart from seasonal hay fever) and didn't think about health at all. You don't when you are young. Sickness is something that happens to other people. Then, after my mother passed away, I came across an article explaining RA responds well to diet. This was the first time I had heard this. I investigated further. At first, curious, then appalled, finally angry, when I discovered Rheumatoid Arthritis is curable, without NSAIDs, Methotrexate, steroids and gold injections, and my mother need not have suffered the terrible end she did. I wanted to know why Doctors did not know about this, when it came from their own literature? Why dietary therapies were not being applied to RA sufferers in hospitals? Why Doctors did not know about natural methods of healing. Juice and water fasts, raw food diets, hydrotherapy and so on. At Antarana, my Wellness Retreat, I see RA symptoms disappear within 14 days, just through dietary change.

Then I discovered a world I had no idea existed. A world where Doctors are not allowed to suggest alternatives or deviate from 'Standard Practice', otherwise they can be struck off. A frightening dystopian world, where parents of children with cancer can be jailed, or lose their children to the State if they don't submit them to the violent assault that is chemotherapy, radiation and surgery. Even when their odds of survival from such treatments are virtually zero. A world where the State can kidnap your children for not allowing them to be vaccinated, though they may be healthier than other children, under the invented and false pretext of 'herd immunity'. A world seemingly gone mad, where what was once normal and natural is now labelled 'child abuse'. Where pharmaceutical industry 'robber barons' control medicine, for profit. Not Doctors, for health. I started to dig a little deeper and learned how the health system really works as opposed to how I thought it worked. It is a business run by businessmen and as long as treatments make more money than cures, we will have treatments and no cures. Doctors fight valiantly to save lives. I might have died on two occasions without them. For acute and emergency conditions they are first class. But for chronic and degenerative disorders, 75% of what plagues us, they can do little, only make matters worse. I learned the system is a failure. How That it has been designed to fail. Because if it succeeded, it would put itself out of business. I discovered an unofficial history of medicine, instead of the approved version, which shed more light on why there were no cures. That, when courageous healers dared to cure the sick, the health 'cops', on behalf of the medical 'robbers', would persecute them and suppress knowledge of their methods. Often waiting until the healers had made enough money for the 'smash and grab' to be worthwhile. In the suppressed **1953 Fitzgerald Report** the Chief Investigator did not mince his words...

"Public and private funds have been thrown around like confetti at a country fair to close up and destroy clinics, hospitals, and scientific research laboratories which do not conform to the viewpoint of medical associations."

I found out how promising treatments and natural compounds would never be approved because it takes hundreds of millions of dollars to get them through clinical trials. How natural products cannot be patented. Which means only un-natural molecules are approved, even when known to be less effective and harmful. Then I understood. This is a very exclusive Club, into which only the wealthiest corporations are granted access. There was so much more I did not know. How our present-day health system was created and by which powerful, controlling families. Why fossil-fuel-derived, pharmaceutical 'medicine' came to be so dominant and how chemistry and technology came to trump biology (you may have noticed lately how biology is making a comeback, with 'Bio'-this and 'Bio'-that).

I learned why Cancer treatments have not changed in decades and how cancer charities and pink ribbons are a cynical sham, fleecing the public. They must be, if you think about it. The mandated conventional treatment, for over 60 years, is chemotherapy, radiation and surgery. Or else. Doctors attempting non-mandated methods can be struck off or jailed. This being the case, why do Cancer charities nag the public constantly for donations 'for research'? There has been NO serious investigation into cancer cures at all and certainly not into alternatives. Quite the opposite. Cancer charities work with medical associations to undermine medical schools, hospitals and practitioners, even when they have ample clinical evidence and customer testimonials, showing non-toxic methods have greater therapeutic value than existing treatments. When you start to dig, you discover cancer research is almost always designed to fail.

You learn from people like Ben Goldacre, who wrote 'Bad Pharma', how studies can be rigged and science manipulated, to sell junk food pyramids, junk flu pandemics, junk remedies and to dismiss alternatives. You learn only positive outcomes of trials are published and negative data is buried, so Doctors cannot make decisions on the basis of ALL the evidence. Of the immense damage pharmaceutical drugs cause and the many side effects your Doctor never informed you of. Or learn from Nature, a weekly science journal, how most prescribed drugs do not work for the majority taking them. How only 2%, if that, benefit from taking Statins. Which means 98% are only getting the side effects.

You discover the top 5 drug companies earn more in one year than the whole continent of Africa. That patients get better ON treatment not BECAUSE of treatment. There was so much to take in. Once I started digging I could not stop. Each shocking new revelation chipping away at my childlike trust and naivety regarding Health Care. Or should it be Sickness Care?

I learned I was an entry in an health corporation's balance sheet, generating expected lifetime revenue of $275,000 from medication, for my 'incurable' disease and if, like many patients, I'm taking three or more medicines, what a bonanza for owners and shareholders. That, in the last two years of my life, what was left of my assets, including my home, would be pounced on to pay for cancer treatment or heart by-pass operations. A final mugging by the Corporate State as I passed on. I knew it was true, knowing families thrown out of their homes because a parent, or family member, could not afford health insurance. Or even if they could, were denied by a myriad of exclusions.

I have had a taste of medical racketeering. In an emergency visit to a private hospital, in Thailand, due to food poisoning, it was clear all they cared about was my ability to pay. You could argue this is reasonable. However, when they saw I could, fees were jacked up and suddenly I am pressured to take all kinds of tests and procedures and encouraged to stay 'just a few more days' for 'observation', a euphemism for 'we haven't finished picking your pocket'. After 4 days, I was relieved to escape with the obligatory shopping trolley full of over-priced meds. Thailand's Prime Minister promised to rein in hospital charges after street protests.

All of this is depressing and upsetting and I am well aware people do not like to hear it but I needed to know. Because, by not knowing, I had stayed too long within a system only too happy to keep me sick. Sometimes I wish I had remained ignorant. It is heart-breaking to see millions suffering and dying when their diseases are preventable and can be cured. I have to bring myself back to focusing on the positive. That, whatever happened in the past, and is still happening today, does not have to be our future. Instead of being passive actors in this real-life drama, we can be revolutionaries. The vanguard of a human wave, taking back control of our health and the health of our children. A wave seeking to give medicine back its soul. A wave saying to Medical Authorities, "If you refuse to cure us, step aside while we cure ourselves". Thanks to the internet I discovered my disorders were not 'incurable' after all. Learned healers existed who had cured cancer and heart disease, arthritis and diabetes, depression and anxiety. Today, the same methods that cured my arthritis, years ago, in India, can easily be found, a few mouse-clicks away. I can order Amazonian rain-forest herbs, design my own healing program and source everything I need for it, online. I am in the 'Bypass Age' and, just like water flows around a rock, can bypass all that has failed, and cure myself.

The good news is, if I can do it, so can you.

What's Inside

I cannot know what you already know but if you have made it this far, WELL DONE. You are demonstrating you are serious about resolving your health issues and transforming your life. I understand, when you purchase a book such as this, you are seeking a cure and want to get right to the bit telling you how to achieve it. It should be EASY, needs to work QUICKLY and has to be AFFORDABLE. If you could just pop a pill, or herb, without doing anything else, fantastic! Or ask me to send you the contact details of the Naturopath who confidently stated he could have cured me in 3 days. I promise I will share his cure with you, later.

Our desire for a 'quick fix' is understandable. We have been conditioned, from childhood, to expect it. Unfortunately, reality is not so accommodating. While there are miraculous cures... and I present some in these pages... you have tried the 'magic bullet' approach and it has not worked. You have also tried the herb approach and found it has not worked either. You need to understand, more often than not, you are on the right track but have failed to grasp WHY these methods have not worked. Once you have the key that unlocks the secret of how to use therapies, supplements and so on, they WILL work.

Let me start with what is not in the book. I promised friends I would avoid too much technical detail and medical jargon and keep it simple. There are few technical references. You won't look at them anyway. Academics and professionals, seeking more detail, know where to look. Much of the information I present is in the public domain and can be found with the help of 'Dr Google'.

I explain what is making us sick so we can begin to reverse it. I explain why Doctors cannot cure, so you know it is a dead-end. I recount my own health struggle so you can learn from it. Then explain, in a way that is easy to understand, why the program I used to heal myself has a better chance of success than anything else you may have tried.

"There are two ways to be fooled. One is to believe what isn't true; the other is to refuse to believe what is true."

Soren Kierkergard

Are You Open?

When faced with information contradicting their existing beliefs, 96% of people will resist, while 4% are open. I mention this because your beliefs are going to be challenged, just as mine were. I do not apologize. The scale of sickness in the U.S. and increasingly around the world is a planetary emergency. Unless people are shocked into awareness they will not pay attention, stick to a healing program or change their disease-inducing ways.

It is a sad fact the majority of people prefer comforting lies to unpleasant truths. 'Fluoride is good for your teeth'; 'Saturated fat makes you fat'; 'High cholesterol causes heart attacks'; The Doctor knows best'; 'Alternative medicine is 'quackery''. There are many more but you get the idea. These myths are written to our mental hard drives from an early age and rarely questioned. Yet, when you investigate them, they are quickly revealed as false. The practice of propaganda is to repeat something often enough and loud enough until it becomes 'truth'. Then no-one questions it. If someone does, we think them 'crazy'. A vast number of false beliefs have been firmly implanted into the minds of the populace, via the mass media, over many decades, using fear as the tool.

Fear works. Ask the medical profession. Ask the Cancer Industry, who do not shy away from using fear to drive patients through their doors. Ask the media. One industry insider called regular media fear campaigns, like H1N1, SARS and Ebola, 'cattle drives'. The latest is the Zika virus. I long ago turned off the TV, to tune the political and media fear-mongering cowboys out. My world is a far happier place as a result. Listening to those spreading disinformation, telling me who I am supposed to hate, which peoples our sons in the military are expected to murder, which satanic pop diva, wearing a crucifix while grabbing her crotch, our pre-teen daughters are supposed to emulate, and which blood-drenched Hollywood 'blockbuster' I am supposed to get excited about, is hardly good for my health or peace of mind. Having said that, fear only motivates for a short period. When, what we are being frightened with fails to materialize, people stop caring. Until the next media hobgoblin is unleashed to frighten us once more.

We do not use fear to motivate those who attend our Retreats. We remove it. Progress is your motivation. When you start to feel alive again, when your depression lifts, when you throw open the curtains in the morning and shout to the world... "I FEEEEEL Great!!!" there is no room for fear. It has been replaced with hope and renewal and gratitude. In my experience of yoga, detox and wellness retreats, it takes only 4-5 days to start feeling vital and alive again. Even after decades of feeling awful.

The information I present is, to my knowledge, accurate and up to date. Where possible, figures come from the health industry's own published data. I do not claim my way is the only way. In fact I do not claim it is even MY way. I give credit where it is due and pay homage to the great healers of yesterday and today, whose teachings have stood the test of time and from whom I draw inspiration. Their guidance is badly needed in this horribly corrupt age. If you disagree strongly with anything I present, let me know. If I agree with you, I will make corrections. If some of my information is out of date, or incomplete, likewise. Until then, take what is useful and discard what is not.

Areas addressed in the book:

Why your Doctor will NEVER cure you

Why Alternatives COULD cure but don't

My journey from sickness to health

What you can do to cure yourself

You will find a host of useful insights to help you make better health choices. No need to do as I did, travel the world seeking cures. No need to spend thousands of hours on research, wade through complex technical documents or become frustrated and helpless in the face of constantly changing and contradictory views. Inside, you will find:

Forgotten and suppressed healing knowledge

A simplified view of health

The one step missing that is the KEY to success

A safe, practical program for healing which can be tried at home

By the time you reach the last page, something inside you will have changed. You will have new hope. Will no longer be confused or dependent on others. You will be your own Doctor. By the way. When you choose health over disease, prepare for some attention. People will see the change in you and want to know how you did it!

'The whole aim of practical politics is to keep the populace alarmed (and hence clamorous to be led to safety) by menacing it with an endless series of hobgoblins, all of them imaginary.'

H.L. Mencken

The Health You Deserve

We all deserve a life of glowing health and vitality, free from pain and sickness. Whether in Body, Mind or Spirit. It is our birthright. To be happy. To be at peace. To enjoy a long, healthy existence on this beautiful planet. To love ourselves, our families and our fellow man. To pass away peacefully in our sleep. Such a life is attainable if we manage our lives wisely and live in accordance with natural laws.

Unfortunately, most of us are set for a very different experience. A host of mental and physical maladies have befallen mankind, like Biblical plagues. Diseases and disorders I never heard of as a child are now 'incurable' epidemics. The number of these conditions is staggering and getting worse. There are around 80 Auto-Immune disorders, 200 types of Arthritis, 200 different Cancers and over 300 Psychiatric disorders. In the U.S. half of all men will get Cancer and a third of women. When I was young it was 1 in 25. 100 years ago, it was 1 in 1000. Coronary artery disease is the No.1 killer, yet it barely existed before 1900. 1 BILLION people globally - 70% of Americans, 66% of Britons and 63% of Australians are overweight or obese. Obesity rates in Australia are climbing faster than anywhere else in the world. The cost to society of obesity-linked disease, is staggering.

Modern medicine does brilliant things with Acute and Emergency care. Yet, for Chronic and Degenerative disorders such as Cancer, Heart and Cerebrovascular Disease (stroke), which cause 75% of deaths in industrialized nations, it is a colossal failure. Millions are set to be tortured, scarred, mutilated, poisoned and burned by well-meaning but ignorant medical doctors, attempting to relieve suffering, until they are finally rejected and sent home to die. Think I am exaggerating? In 2013, the National Cancer Institute admitted two important cancers; early stage breast cancer and prostate cancer, were NOT cancers after all but harmless lesions. Over a 30 year period, 1.3 million women had been subjected to some combination of either mastectomy, lumpectomy, radiation, and chemotherapy. Many more were filled with fear and dread. Who knows how many new cancers these interventions created? The same applies to thousands of men, wrongly diagnosed with prostate cancer. It should have been front page news, worldwide.

This appalling harm and embarrassing re-assessment would not be necessary with safer, non-toxic, non-invasive alternatives. In the U.S., Dr Dean Ornish has proven his program to reverse heart disease, using diet, stress reduction and exercise, works. Patients can be out of danger within a month. Yet, a friend who recently underwent triple-bypass surgery, allowing himself to believe he was getting 'brand new plumbing', is carrying livid scars on his leg and chest and has to spend a year recovering. He had never heard of Dean Ornish or his program.

Nor had his Doctor ever suggested it. Why? If someone asked me if I prefer 12 months on a healing diet or have a surgeon saw open my chest, rip out a vein from my leg, plunge a knife into my heart, with the possibility I might die on the operating table, I think I might like a stab at the diet. In what way is undergoing major surgery better than a year eating healthy food, exercising and reducing stress, which will put me out of danger, restore ALL of my circulatory system, resolve other disorders I may have and renew my love of life? What makes the Doctor's failure-to-inform all the more reprehensible is studies show heart-bypass surgery and the insertion of stents does little to extend the lives of patients. I suspect the good Doctor is either ignorant of the Ornish protocol; he believes patients will not follow it; heart surgeons would lose their jobs or, dare I suggest, surgery is far more profitable than this natural method, given to Dr Ornish by an Indian Swami.

My mother spent her last two years suffering what I can only describe as medieval medical cruelty, due to chronic Rheumatoid Arthritis. The Doctors were conscientious and heroic but limited to pain management, which devastated her body more than the disease. Appalled at her suffering, I asked if there was anything else the family could try? The Doctors said 'No'. I did not know then but I certainly know now, they were wrong. After one too many trips to intensive care, she was finally put out of her misery, with an overdose of morphine.

What has happened to healing? Where is the effort to cure disease? We are supposed to have a Health system not a Disease Management system. When you only manage symptoms and make no attempt to address underlying cause, are you even a Doctor? Doctors may have abdicated their responsibility to cure but they can only work within the boundaries set for them, using the tools and medical education they are provided with. If a Doctor's education is narrow and limited, so will be his practice. It does not matter how brilliant they are... and many Doctors ARE technically brilliant doctors are incentivized and directed to treat and not cure. To dismiss alternatives, not investigate and embrace them. Doctors are woefully ignorant of how to cure. Sadly, it is the nature of ignorance the ignorant are unaware they are ignorant! How can a supposedly intelligent human being, whose remit is to save life, embrace and defend a system which kills and injures millions, regards 75% of what ails mankind as 'incurable', then mocks and denigrates alternatives that injure and kill no-one? The medical profession's callous arrogance beggars belief. Which is why millions are voting with their feet.

Remember when they used to give drugs for temporary relief? In the space of a decade society shifted to taking them for life. Who benefits from this? Well, the Doctor is happy. He is kept employed and rewarded. Health Corporations are happy, their owners reap stupendous profits. More so when diseases progress to Cancer, heart disease and severe disability (patients pay more when they think they are going to die). Politicians are happy. They receive their stock options, 'campaign contributions' and lucrative seats on Boards of Directors. The media are happy, raking in millions from corporate promotions and advertising. Society in general benefits from more hospitals and jobs in health care. Sickness is a huge generator of economic activity. Why would any of those benefiting from this wish to see a healthier society? How about you? Are you happy paying for your Doctor's BMW while you struggle to afford a wheelchair and are directed to take synthetic, toxic chemicals, for the rest of your days? Pills which will never cure, only suppress your symptoms and prevent you taking steps to heal yourself. Let's not kid ourselves. Until you address the underlying cause of your disease, you are not getting better.

Doctors tell you to watch your diet, yet know little of nutrition. Millions have become sick and fat, following government Food Pyramid guidelines, heavily influenced by the meat and dairy industries. Despite their infatuation with science, Doctors do not know how the body works. If they did, they would not be dying from the same diseases we do. If Doctors knew how to prevent or cure Cancer, they would not get Cancer, and if they did, would be able to cure it in themselves. But they do and they can't. So why would anyone with Cancer, seeking a cure, go to a conventional Doctor? For ANY 'incurable' disease? Patients, frustrated with Doctors failure to cure, increasingly look elsewhere, turning toward CAM (Complementary or Alternative Methods). Some Doctors, too. The coming together of conventional and alternative systems is known as Integrative Medicine. Functional Medicine is another development. 40% of patients in the U.S. are enjoying safe, non-toxic, non-invasive treatments which support the body, not burden it. Examples are Acupuncture, Homeopathy, Osteopathy, Chiropractic and Herbalism. These methods can be helpful. Unfortunately, for reasons I explain, they rarely cure chronic and degenerative disorders.

In Germany, German Biological Medicine has grown out of Doctors' greater freedom to innovate. This highly complex system draws on several different methods of healing: - ancient, modern and alternative. There is no attachment to a particular modality, nor are practitioners required to stay within rigidly imposed boundaries. This approach makes perfectly good sense. I adopted a simpler version to cure my own disorders.

What about pills? A multi-billion dollar, over-the-counter (OTC) supplements industry has grown up to meet consumer demand for 'instant fixes' but they are invariably useless, if not completely fraudulent. As a result we end up returning to our Doctors, still sick, poorer in pocket and with a skeptical attitude toward alternatives.

Then there is the most important factor in WHY we get sick and how we can recover. We all make excuses but let's face it. The reason we are sick is due to the choices WE make, each and every day. Every time we choose to consume junk food, sweet biscuits or sweetened sodas, we are creating imbalance, a nutritional deficit and disease within our bodies. Every time we fail to exercise, we create stagnation and toxic accumulation. Every time we are rude, negative, angry or fearful, deceitful, lacking in love, compassion and consideration for ourselves and our fellow man, we are creating conditions for psychological and physical disease to take hold and dare I suggest, in this God-less age, spiritual death. Given a choice between fresh fruit and a sticky bun, we turn our noses up at the fruit and opt for the bun. The fruit is building health ("An apple a day") while the bun is building disease. We choose disease, even when we know the fruit builds health.

For any biological species this is insanity. We are committing suicide with our forks and do not seem to know or care. Not only are we killing ourselves but also our children. Guaranteeing, in them, the same chronic disorders we are suffering. Remember when they called it adult-onset diabetes? No more. Now babies are born with diabetes. Unfortunately, too many parents are psychologically divorced from actions which harm their children. In and out of the womb.

What about Mental Health? The numbers are staggering. 25% of Americans have some kind of mental disorder. 1 in 4 of the population. How many of these 'disorders' are due to a deficiency of Zoloft, or Prozac, or Xanax, or Ativan? None. 6 million children in America (and increasingly in the UK), who should be outside, climbing trees, are forced to sit in grey, concrete, confinement centres, known as schools. When they show signs of boredom and restlessness, they are given Ritalin (methylphenidate), classified by the Drug Enforcement Administration as a Schedule II narcotic. The same classification as cocaine, morphine and amphetamines. I thought we had a 'War ON Drugs' not a 'War OF Drugs'. These children are being raised in poverty, their bodies and minds poisoned by vaccines, chemical sugars and subversive messages to 'do what you want'. Have you seen a children's cartoon lately? How, cynically, cartoon characters like 'Spongebob Squarepants' are used to plant bad behaviour and 'attitude' in the minds of the young. Messages to defy parents. To demand what is bad for them. Every cartoon filled with burgers, hot dogs, sodas and ice-cream. The brainwashing is not even subtle. It's the same with infant educational material. The effect on developing minds and bodies, from this psychological assault, is devastating. It has been going on for decades. Creating sick, addicted parents who produce sick, addicted children. Caring parents are cynically undermined by the corporate mass media instilling 'needs' and 'wants' in the young, for profit. Their health be damned.

Humanity is being flushed down the evolutionary toilet. We are the most diseased generation in the history of mankind. The scale of disease is such it can no longer be called an accident. In every aspect of our lives today we see "garbage in, garbage out". The solutions we are presented with do not work and, on closer examination, are crafted to do even more damage, while presented as 'advances'. Orwell's Doublespeak and the 'Big Lie' evident, every time you turn on the news. Do you think President Obama's much-vaunted 'Personalized Medicine' initiative is going to cure anyone? Genetics is only one facet of who we are. Perhaps 1% in significance. Genetics gives us the blueprint for building a body but who is the project manager? Who gives it life? Who or what decides whether a gene is turned on or off? What does genetics have to do with someone who cannot afford to eat healthy food and has no choice but to purchase nuggets, sodas and fries? What does the science of genetics have to do with how we think or what we believe; the decision to exercise or flop on the sofa; to be violent or peaceful? Half of America has diabetes, 75% are obese, and we are focusing on genes, instead of locking up and confiscating the wealth of those who have caused this.

It is a sick civilization which allows the poisoning of hundreds of millions so a handful of predatory 'Masters of the Universe' can enjoy obscene riches and lord it over us? Why isn't the money being spent on genetics, warmongering, and bailing out corrupt bankers, used to provide us with uncontaminated soil, healthy food and decent housing? Genetics is going to make already-wealthy owners even richer and you can be sure who will be paying the price. You and I. A conscience-less criminal class, dressed in suits and ties, is showing the rest of the world what lies in store for them.

Do not misunderstand. There are cures out there. I am going to tell you about them. There are healers out there. I have encountered them. Compassionate men and women who have taken patients, sent home by hospitals to die, and cured them using simple, safe, natural methods. The word 'incurable' not in their vocabulary. Dr Max Gerson and his inspirational daughter, Charlotte, have been healing Cancer, heart disease and other serious conditions, since the 1930s. Dr Gerson cured Nobel Prize winner Albert Schweitzer of Type II Diabetes, and his wife of tuberculosis, at a time when TB was taking thousands of lives and considered 'incurable'. Schweitzer said of Max Gerson…

"…I see in him one of the most eminent geniuses in the history of medicine."

Praise indeed. Yet why had I never heard of him and why was I not taught about him in school and why are Doctors not offering us the same cure for diabetes Albert Schweitzer received? When you read Max Gerson's Wikipedia page, as people researching will, it is so damning you want to lock him up and throw away the key. The message is clear. The man is a charlatan, his methods 'quackery' and just in case you were thinking of giving his 'unproven' ideas a go, doing so might kill you. One might wonder, if Dr Gerson was curing diabetes, tuberculosis and cancers when other Doctors couldn't, who exactly the 'quacks' are? Hit-pieces such as this are standard fare on mainstream sites, which condemn the speck (usually exaggerated) in an Alternative's eye, while ignoring the plank in its own. When you have seen enough of them, you recognize the tactics used to discourage you from moving to the competition. Unfortunately, too many people, including Doctors, believe what they read.

Twenty years ago I won a national Information Technology Award. Next to the birth of my children it was my proudest moment. Head-hunters called me, offering lucrative positions. My financial future was secure. I turned them down. Partly out of loyalty to my employer but principally because I was 'burnt-out'; taking anti-depressants just to be able to sleep. This is something I rarely see talked about. The effects of chronic illness on families. On relationships and budgets. On carers and careers. I have just come off the phone to a lovely lady, whose father is in intensive care, with major health problems and no insurance. The family have expended their life savings on medical bills and are going deep into debt to save him. With each Intensive Care intervention, the debts mount. This, when she has recently undergone a double mastectomy for breast cancer. My heart goes out to her and her family. The effects of sudden and serious illness can be catastrophic.

I wish my mother had known about Dr Max Gerson. I wish my father, who died at 54, from diabetes-related heart failure, had known about Dr Dean Ornish. I wish I had known of Linus Pauling and Dr Abram Hoffer who, 50 years ago, were using nutrition to cure psychiatric and physical disorders. I wish I had discovered earlier, the fascinating, traditional Ayurvedic healer who, in a small clinic, in an Indian backwater, cured my arthritis. Most of all, I wish our doctors knew how to cure. It would have saved me years of physical and mental torment, the breakup of my family and the end of my career.

Someone I do know about is Dr Richard Schulze, Naturopath and Master Herbalist. Richard secretly healed patients for twenty years before he was forced to stop practicing. He believes absolutely… "THERE ARE NO INCURABLE DISEASES". This colossus of natural healing would see patients four months after they were given only two months to live… the worst of the worst… and cure them. His 'Save Your Life' video series is a veritable treasure chest of natural healing techniques used to cure cancers and chronic disorders. Not everyone cares for Richard's outspoken honesty and 'radical' methods but there is no doubting his ability to heal, his vast experience and his power to motivate. He would be the first person I would ask for, if seriously ill. A less extreme colossus is Linus Pauling, winner of two Nobel's and one of the founders of Orthomolecular Medicine. Wiki says of Dr Pauling…

'...one of the most influential chemists in history and ranks among the most important scientists of the 20th century.'

Praise indeed. Linus Pauling surely knows what he is talking about. So I bring up the Wiki page on Orthomolecular Medicine. What does it say?

'...a form of food faddism and even quackery.'

'...untested'

Rounding off the mugging,

'...some vitamins have been linked to increased risk of cancer and death.'

Goodness. Who would try high dose vitamin therapy after reading that? But hold on a moment. Read the last sentence carefully,

'...some vitamins have been linked to increased risk...'

It is clever and misleading. What does 'linked' mean, exactly and who linked it? Did they use natural, whole vitamins? Most high street vitamins are synthetic, inorganic fractions of vitamins. Notice they don't say exactly which vitamins, so you will likely avoid them all. 'Increased risk' is not quantified. Is it major or insignificant? Let's try this, ourselves. Imagine someone is killed in a collision with a truck and the driver had fallen asleep at the wheel. It happens. The media have received orders from above to smear a vitamin which is becoming too popular. So, they report the incident as,

'A truck driver, who fell asleep at the wheel, killing an innocent pedestrian, had been taking Vitamin C.'

The implication, clearly, is the accident was somehow related to Vitamin C. How much greater would be the emotional impact on the viewer if he had killed a bus full of handicapped schoolchildren? We could make this game of linking a little more interesting. Most high street Vitamin C is derived from genetically modified corn. Thus, the gutter press headline becomes,

'Truck of Death linked to GM corn!'

See how it works? If you wish to sew doubt in the public mind, simply 'link' to the practitioner, method, or product, you seek to undermine. By the way. The leading brand of vitamins in the U.S. is called Centrum. Laboratory analysis recently found Centrum vitamins contain GMO, Food Dyes & Toxic Chemicals. Be aware most High Street 'vitamins' are synthetic, inorganic and not the whole vitamin. Because there are no set standards, or levels, for multivitamins, it would not surprise me if someone DID sicken or die from taking them. When the media report on those 'dangerous' or 'deadly' vitamins, they are probably referring to synthetic vitamins. Whole, natural vitamins do not cause harm.

In my opinion, Linus Pauling, Max and Charlotte Gerson, Richard Schulze, Dean Ornish and others are heroes, meriting the highest accolades for the contributions they have made to healing. Instead, they remain largely unknown, their methods given no official acknowledgment, except to undermine practitioner or therapy. It is almost impossible to find anyone curing cancer, in western industrialized nations. They operate in secret, or are forced to practice abroad. If a cancer, herb or product is successful against cancer, but not approved by Medical Associations or the FDA, practitioners are shut down. Competition will not be tolerated. Practitioners who are able to bring about healing are, instead, limited to teaching, writing books (like this) and selling supplements. There is no freedom of choice. Only medical dictatorship.

When I fired my doctor and traveled to other countries, seeking cures for my own 'incurable' disorders, so impressed was I by the healers I met and so astounded by the simplicity of their methods, I decided to learn how they did it, so I could help myself and others. Now, because there is such great need in society, it is time to add my voice to those who have gone before and share my knowledge with you. You need to know what you are doing wrong, so you can put it right. You need to learn to be your own Doctor because YOU are the one who makes all the choices. Nobody else. If you do not learn how to take care of yourself and your loved ones... knowledge now vital... you are lost. We all are. My heart goes out to those who have searched in vain for help. Who have listened to 'expert' opinion and abandoned hope, believing nothing can be done.

DO NOT BELIEVE THEM!

Recovering one's health does not have to be complicated. All you need is a clear understanding of what steps to take and the will and motivation, not only to get started, but to succeed. To end all those years where you have said to yourself, day after day, week after week, month after month, "Tomorrow. I will definitely start tomorrow".

Do you tell yourself, "It is too difficult"? Are you frustrated and discouraged by previous failure? Banish these thoughts, look in the mirror and ask yourself a question.

"DO I WANT TO LIVE OR DO I WANT TO DIE?"

If you want to live, the knowledge and ideas in this book will help you. If you want to die, please continue on your way and may whichever God you worship, bless your journey.

You DO want to live, don't you?

That's why you bought this book.

"Do not let either the medical authorities or the politicians mislead you. Find out what the facts are and make your own decisions about how to live a happy life and how to work for a better world."

Linus Pauling

Approach with Care

The Internet is the new enlightenment. Unlike my parent's generation, who received information through tightly controlled news outlets, the internet presents us with a great deal more information, good and bad. Enabling us to make informed choices. It is a marvellous healing tool, relieving symptoms of ignorance in all those who use it, wisely. Sadly, it has its downside, revealing things we really wish we didn't know. If you have spent time online, searching for health solutions, you will almost certainly have encountered the unpleasant side of research. A veritable army, some paid, await the unwary. Their remit? To dissuade the public from trying alternatives and keep them in the conventional, corporate-medicine fold. Armed with the 3D's, 'Disrupt, Defame and Deter', they are a menace to open discussion. You may have encountered them. Natural healing sites; personal or natural health blogs; health-related Facebook groups; internet community forums. They are easy to identify. I used to be drawn into argument with them. Now my time is better spent on those who have ears to hear.

Also to be approached with care, are impressive-sounding Consumer Protection websites and 'Scientific' health blogs. They like nothing better than sticking a scientific boot into 'quackery'. Most are industry fronts, using deception and deflection to mislead. What do I mean? An example of deception is when a site or individual says an alternative therapy, or product, has not been properly tested. They use terms like:

"No trials". "Unscientific". "Unproven".

The implication, of course, is this is bad. Like Pavlovian pups, trained to respond to a negative stimulus, we steer clear and return to the conventional fold. We have been deceived in three ways.

1. Omission. What they don't tell you is natural methods or compounds will never be tested by orthodox medicine because they cannot be patented. Nor is the present system able to test natural methods. There are too many variables. (More on this later).

2. Lies. Natural healing has been tested over hundreds, if not thousands of years. Personal testimony, case studies, trial and error and simple observation are evidence. Studies do exist. You just do not know where to find them.

3. Deflection. Whatever you accuse the other guy of doing is what YOU are doing. We see this all the time in politics. In medicine, accuse your competition of not having tested their products, even though your own products and methods are largely untested. The Randomized Control Trial (RCT) is a relatively recent

innovation. 100 years of prior medical practice has yet to be subjected to RCTs. It won't be. It is too expensive to do so and estimates suggest at least 50% of existing medical practice would fail clinical trials. While individual drugs may have been tested, most do not undergo long-term safety tests. Combinations of pharmaceutical drugs, which many of us now take, more so the elderly, have never been tested. Likewise, thousands of synthetic chemicals on the market. In other words:

"No trials". "Unscientific". "Unproven".

Then there is the criminal practice of physicians routinely writing "off-label" prescriptions. Treating conditions with drugs for which there is no official approval.

"No trials". "Unscientific". "Unproven".

IBM has some impressive, futuristic, online medical software, called Watson Health. On its web page, right now, a video introduction informs us of the following:

'50% of medical decisions are not evidence-based.'

'Medical data is expected to double every 75 days until 2020'

It's somewhat ironic to observe medical professionals parroting the meme "Alternatives lack evidence", when IBM informs us there is little substantive evidence for at least half of what Doctors do. I say 'at least' because in 2011, Scientific American reported:

'Only a fraction of what physicians do is based on solid evidence from Grade-A randomized, controlled trials; the rest is based instead on weak or no evidence and on subjective judgment. When scientific consensus exists on which clinical practices work effectively, physicians only sporadically follow that evidence correctly.'

A 'fraction' sounds a lot less than half. Sites like 'Quackwatch' are nowhere to be seen when it comes to the failings of corporate medicine. If they were to shine a light on them in the same way they do alternatives there would be a revolution in the morning. They won't, of course. That's not their purpose. I sympathize with Doctors who are as overwhelmed by information as we are. They need 3 brains to process it all.

There is a major issue with 'Standard Practice'. This is official guidance or directives on the best treatment for a particular disease or disorder. Doctors are forced to apply treatments they know to be harmful, or useless, on pain of losing their license to practice. Allopathic medicine can take a decade or more to change its procedures or practices, in the face of advances or adverse outcomes. Which means surgeries and treatments are being conducted that are outdated, known to be of little value, or cause harm. 'Standard Practice' is the Medical Associations' method of forcing conformity and shutting out any other possibility.

Care must be exercised when encountering zealots. These are people who have never tried an alternative therapy in their lives, know nothing about them yet howl with outrage if you suggest they have merit. Their attitude is ignorant and irrational. If my car stops working and I take it to a garage and they cannot fix it, I take it somewhere else. People would think me silly NOT to. Yet, if I go to my Doctor and he can't fix my body or mind and I go elsewhere, I am committing a cardinal sin. It does not matter to these people their product is 'not fit for purpose' and conventional medicine doesn't cure. It does not matter my body and health choices are none of their damn business. I must stick with what doesn't work and not go near those 'dangerous' alternatives (they like to turn this around). Even when you contrast the shocking numbers killed and injured by modern medicine, with the total lack of harm from natural or alternative methods, they still fume and fulminate. What kind of dysfunctional thinking is willing to see human beings die rather than allow them access to safer alternatives which may work? Oncologists KNOW chemotherapy does not work on most cancers, injures or kills millions, yet apply the treatment anyway. How is this not a criminal act?

I understand why Doctors think like this. 12 years of medical and ongoing education, influenced by drug companies and medical associations, drums into you alternative medicine is 'quackery' and practitioners are 'kooks'. Scientific medicine is 'state of the art', while old medicine is superstition and blood-letting and medicine-men with bones through their noses. That those cured without the intervention of a Medical Doctor are 'spontaneous remissions' and not cured as a result of their own efforts. Alternatives are 'dangerous' because they seduce you away from 'proper' medicine, which will keep you alive, even if it cannot cure you. Faced with this level of indoctrination, you are guaranteed to be met with scepticism and hostility.

An example of Big Pharma's influence over Doctors is the Merck Manual, otherwise known as 'The Doctor's Bible'. It is produced, not by Doctors but a drug company. Rest assured (cough... cough...) there is no conflict of interest. Merck is the drug company which produced Vioxx, estimated to have triggered the deaths of 120,000 victims before it was withdrawn. Merck knew Vioxx doubled the risk of heart attacks, yet hid the fact. A deeper investigation of the scandal revealed a variety of criminal and unethical practices by the company, including the intimidation of investigators. Merck is likely to be involved in a bigger scandal over Gardasil, a vaccine supposedly preventing cervical cancer, which two of its leading Doctors have suggested will eventually become recognized as "the greatest medical scandal of all time". Dr. Bernard Dalbergue denounced its approval and continued use, claiming 'everyone' involved with it knows it is completely worthless. Damage inflicted by Gardasil? Sudden death, paralysis, encephalitis, Guillain-Barre syndrome and a host of other ailments. Merck also publishes the 'Veterinarian Bible', using the same marketing model to push vaccines and drugs on our pets.

I mustn't leave out the patients. If you have been taking Statins for 15 years, all the while believing they are protecting you, and someone points out you have been misled, you are going to experience some serious indigestion and fight to defend your belief. Typically, by 'shooting the messenger.' My older guests and callers are like this. They were raised to be trusting of the State. They cannot believe the medical industry would lie or knowingly cause harm. They come around eventually, since its failings are increasingly obvious to everyone.

Whatever happened to 'evidence-based medicine'? One of the most blindingly obvious studies to conduct is to compare disease-rates between those who have been vaccinated and those who haven't. Yet, when Congressman Bill Posey questioned the CDC at an **Autism Congressional hearing** in November 2012, the CDC admitted they had never conducted a study in the U.S. comparing vaccinated with unvaccinated children. How difficult is it to get all Doctors, or even a sample of Doctors, to submit the health records of each and every child vaccinated and have rates of asthma, allergies, autism, etc.. compared with the unvaccinated? They have had decades to do this. With everything now entered into computers, it should be easy to obtain the necessary data. Longitudinal studies, using questionnaires, have been conducted in New Zealand and Germany, showing a 5x greater occurrence of common disorders in vaccinated children, than unvaccinated. Official studies conducted in the U.S.?

"No trials". "Unscientific". "Unproven".

"Why Am I Sick, Doc?"

"Why am I sick, Doc?"

"It's Genetic", says the Conventional Doctor.

"Leaky Gut", says the Alternative practitioner.

What a great way to answer the question. Instead of saying, "I have no idea", practitioners make something up. You can understand why. We demand to know what is wrong with us and expect Doctors to have the answer. It used to be believed our genes determined whether we would fall ill and there was pretty much nothing we could do about it. We could lead a healthy life and still get sick. Our genetic blueprint could not be changed. That was the prevailing wisdom. Now we know genes can be switched on and off. This is called gene expression, the science of 'Epigenetics'. What switches them on or off? Lifestyle. The choices we make every day.

Dr James Chestnut, a popular speaker on health matters, provides a neat analogy of how suspect the "It's genetic" answer is. How many times have we seen rivers, lakes and oceans, heavily polluted by oil or chemical spills, with millions of dead and dying birds, fish and seals washed up on the shoreline? Imagine the Health Sector, as it is today, springing into action. Pharmaceutical drugs would be tossed into the water and mini hospitals set up on the shores of lakes, using tiny tools to cut out tumours and body parts, before the birds and fish die. Eminent doctors, faced with this tide of dying wildlife, announce, "It's genetic."

Now apply the same scenario to us. We are 100lbs overweight, with high blood pressure, high blood sugar, high cholesterol, cancer, heart disease, diabetes, digestive disorders and lung problems. Caused by toxic food, toxic relationships, a lack of exercise and a poisoned environment and your Doctor says, "It's genetic."

This is a mutually satisfying game to play. The Doctor maintains an aura of competence. The patient goes home, does not have to make any lifestyle changes, tells everyone they are not responsible for their disease, can do nothing about it, then happily tucks into a box of donuts. Why would Doctors bother with cures if they believe your disease is genetic? Why would you change your disease-inducing ways if you believe the same?

Symptoms of 'Leaky Gut', or Candida overgrowth, are so varied you can understand why alternative practitioners diagnose it. The diagnosis does have some merit. Hippocrates said, "All disease begins in the gut". Many people are suffering digestive disorders as our food becomes more toxic. However, 'Leaky Gut' does appear to be reached for a little too often.

The famous Mayo brothers said the average medical doctor gets only 20% of their diagnoses right. 30% of misdiagnosis results in death or serious injury. Alternative practitioners focussing on symptoms are even worse. Hardly surprising, when so many of our symptoms are vague. Instead of saying they do not know, practitioners diagnose a disorder with many symptoms. If you wish to recover from your disease, do not accept this. You are sick because the choices you make have upset the natural balance within your body. You are sick because you have been building disease and not health, violating Nature's Laws. You are sick because you have handed over responsibility for your health and the health of your children to someone who doesn't know you. You are sick because you have forgotten how to take care of yourself.

In 2013, the **U.S. National Institute of Health (NIH)** reported:

'The United States is among the wealthiest nations in the world, but it is far from the healthiest. For many years, Americans have been dying at younger ages than people in almost all other high-income countries. This health disadvantage prevails even though the U.S. spends far more per person on health care than any other nation'.

For life expectancy, obesity, diabetes, heart disease, COPD (lung disorders), HIV and AIDS, drug deaths and sexually transmitted diseases, America ranked, or came close to ranking, the sickest country out of 17 high-income nations. A staggering 60 million adult Americans have been diagnosed with a mental disorder. The United Kingdom is not far behind. Poor health was no longer occurring toward the end of people's lives, when one might expect it but throughout their lives.

Top reasons presented why so many Americans were sick:

Too many calories

Inadequate Health Care

Poverty, especially child poverty

Lack of exercise

Drug abuse

Poor education

In truth, there were so many reasons it would have been easier to say 'almost everything'. America's health has been deteriorating at an alarming pace. 133 million Americans have at least one chronic disorder. 45% of the population have 'incurable' diseases like cancer, heart disease, asthma, arthritis and diabetes. The prescribing rate for drugs in the U.S. has gone up 55x since the 1960's and keeps increasing. This steep incline shows those suffering chronic conditions are not recovering but staying chronic. The NIH report concluded that, unless action was taken to improve matters, levels of illness in the U.S. would only get worse.

Running briefly through the NIH list:

Too Many Calories

I call these 'Diseases of The Fork'. Either 'diseases of affluence', from eating too much rich food, or 'diseases of poverty', from eating low quality food. World-wide, 60% of all deaths are diet-related.

Inadequate Health Care

Access to high quality treatment is limited to those who can afford it. Remote areas and crime-ridden inner cities struggle to attract quality, medical staff. Alternative health solutions are not allowed to compete. A system which does not take prevention seriously and fails to address underlying cause is clearly a failure.

Diseases of Poverty

'Social inequity kills at an alarming rate' WHO 2009. Malnourishment, environmental and financial stress; poor hygiene; dangerous or dirty occupations. A lack of access to health care, leading to higher rates of infant and childhood illnesses and higher mortality rates; exposure to household chemicals; hidden or untreated infection.

Lack of Exercise

Physical inactivity is a primary cause of at least 35 chronic diseases. Circulation is reduced, you lack proper oxygenation; acid and other wastes are not excreted efficiently; muscles waste and you are not burning excess calories. As actress Helen Hayes informs us... "If You Rest, You Rust!"

Drug Abuse

I regard any substance you are addicted to, or using to self-tranquillize, as a 'drug'. That includes food, alcohol, smoking, gambling, sex, pharmaceutical and street drugs and even addiction to stress itself ('adrenaline-junkie').

Poor Education

A lack of general education, including sex education. The less well educated are more likely to be taken in by marketing tricks, pseudo-science, dubious and unnecessary medical procedures, and media fear-mongering. If Knowledge=Power, then a lack of knowledge makes the poor power-less.

Unmentioned Causes of Disease

Lack of Breast-Feeding

Numerous studies strongly indicate significantly decreased risks of infection, allergy, asthma, arthritis, diabetes, obesity, cardiovascular disease, and various cancers in both childhood and adulthood, for those who were breast-fed. Protective elements in breast milk are not found in infant formula.

Natural Childbirth

During natural child-birth, new-borns pass close to the anus, picking up important antibodies which strengthen the immune system.

'Electrosmog'

Biological effects of electro-magnetic and wireless radiation surrounding all electrical devices, power lines, home wiring, mobile phones, radio, TV and WiFi. Leading to cancers, hyperactivity, concentration problems, anxiety, irritability, disorientation, distracted behaviour, sleep disorders and headaches.

Heavy Metal Poisoning

The accumulation of heavy metals, in toxic amounts, in the soft tissues of the body, such as Aluminium, Mercury, Fluoride, Arsenic, Lead, Cadmium, Uranium and others. All have been linked to serious illness.

Iatrogenesis

Iatrogenesis is the intervention of a Doctor, which can have a beneficial or deleterious effect on a patient. Sometimes called 'Death by Doctor', Millions have died, will die, and suffer serious adverse effects of botched or unnecessary surgery, drug side effects, incorrect prescribing, and misdiagnoses.

America fares particularly badly with over-medication. The U.S. has 5% of the global population yet consumes 97% of global pharmaceutical output. At any one time 70% of the population are taking one medication, with 50% taking two or more. What impact on America's health and life expectancy does this consumption have? A clue can be found in the 1974 Helsinki Business Study. Research, over 15 years, compared two groups with similar health issues. The first group saw a Doctor once per year, received no medicines and weren't expected to follow lifestyle advice. The second group were placed on a regimen of beta-blockers, antihypertensive and cholesterol meds. Standard treatment for cardiovascular disease. Unexpectedly, the numbers who died were 4x higher in the treated, than the untreated. This completely shattered conventional wisdom. If similar outcomes apply to other disorders, then the more pharmaceutical medication a society consumes, the sicker it becomes. Isn't this exactly what we are seeing?

Vaccines

When compiling a list of reasons we are so sick, it is impossible to exclude vaccination. The subject tends to inspire strong feelings in people one way or the other. Having conducted the research, rather than simply parroting official pronouncements, there is no doubt in my mind vaccines are a major cause of chronic disease. More in the chapter, 'What Price Prevention?'

Depression

30% of the population will suffer from severe anxiety and depression at some stage in their lives, starting young, often after unmanaged family and social stress. Many have more than one disorder. Modern life is all about 24/7 living and stress (keeping up, getting ahead, material wealth) with less and less time to relax. Over 1/3rd of the population who suffer from stress and stress-related diseases are unaware of its causes. Causes of sickness in society, at the macro level, are easy to see and relatively easy to solve. Each of the aforementioned causes can be reversed. Improve food, environment and wealth disparity and end the overuse of chemicals and medicines. Support the family. Provide quality education instead of 'dumbing down' our children (What on earth is the Kardashians?!) If the will were there, governments would address these problems at source, instead of trying to monetize and criminalize individual behaviour. 'Carbon Cops' arresting the public for using a toaster, while Corporations swap massive pollution for a rain-forest in Botswana and STILL pollute, is barmy and unjust.

At the micro (individual) level, solving health problems becomes a little more complex. Yes, we can exercise more, grow our own fruit and veg, recycle, be kinder to each other and ourselves, form cooperatives and shop at farmers markets. In the 'Bypass Age', people are increasingly doing these things. However, urban dwellers do not have this possibility and most cannot afford it. There will be little change to the nation's health until the food and water, provided to our cities, improves.

Unsurprisingly, corporate and military contamination of air, food and water was missing from the report.

Suppressing Symptoms CAUSES Disease

The concept of suppression is well understood in Psychology. We are encouraged to explore our deepest hurts and fears in order to release them. Not 'bottle up' our feelings. Haven't we all encountered someone who keeps it all inside until they explode with rage or violence? Suppression is understood in cancer, where emotional healing is an important part of cancer recovery. It is also understood in natural healing systems like Ayurveda. We have 13 natural urges: The urge to sleep, cry, sneeze, breathe, belch, yawn, vomit, eat, drink, urinate, ejaculate, defecate and flatulate. If you suppress any of these urges there are consequences. For example: suppressing the urge to sleep can lead to insomnia.

Why, then, does modern medicine suppress the body's natural efforts to throw off disease? If you are in pain, the body is telling you something is wrong. If you suppress your pain, there is STILL something wrong, only the pain is no longer there, nagging you to do something about it. The body creates a fever to kill off invading pathogens and even cancer cells. It creates diarrhoea to clean out your 'pipework', flush out worms or parasites and combat self-poisoning (known as 'auto-intoxication') caused by constipation or dehydration. It creates a head cold to carry mucus and sinus blockage out of the body. A sneeze, or cough, to eject an irritant. These are signs of health not sickness. What does your Doctor or pharmacist do? They disable these attempts to heal. What happens to the pathogen the fever would have burned up? It is now free to penetrate the deeper tissues and organs within the body, triggering chronic disease. Yes, you obtained temporary relief but the Doctor only kicked the can down the road.

Surgeons act similarly. A century ago, medical wisdom decreed certain body parts were superfluous to requirements and surgeons started to cut them out. Appendix, tonsils, gall bladder, spleen, adenoids, foreskins. When your tonsils become inflamed, out comes the scalpel. Why cares about underlying cause? Just take a knife to them and we say, "Thank you". Why? Might there have been something in our diet we were sensitive to and our tonsils were telling us, "Don't eat this". Gluten, or peanuts, or baby formula, or dairy, or tobacco? Now the sentry at your gate has been surgically removed, there are no more warnings.

When your appendix is inflamed, perhaps due to food poisoning, the surgeon makes little attempt to save it. Wouldn't injecting antibiotics directly into the local area resolve both the infection and save the appendix? Why surgically remove it? Your appendix is part of your immune system, making white blood cells and antibodies. It produces certain chemicals which help direct white blood cells to those parts of the body where they are needed the most. Now it has gone, your immune system is weaker for it.

Fevers are not dangerous if you keep a patient hydrated. Cancers in Germany are being treated using Whole Body Hyperthermia, which raises the body's temperature to fever levels. Prostate cancers are being cured using localized high temperatures. Artificial fevers and hydrotherapy were being utilized, successfully, by Priessnitz in the 1820's. Creating artificial fevers is a useful weapon in the natural healing armoury. The 'Cold Sheet Treatment' (part of the 'Incurables' program you will read about later) is one example.

Our bodies are constantly kept in balance. Blood pressure, blood sugar, bodily temperature, hormones, cholesterol, our 'microbiome' and so on. This we call homeostasis. So when a particular parameter consistently exceeds the norm, there is obviously something wrong. If the body is producing excess cholesterol it is doing so for a reason. The 'vitalistic' view is that the body is producing cholesterol to protect arteries from excess acidity, caused by a diet rich in acid-forming foods. It is unnatural for humans to eat such an acidic diet. What do Doctors do? They artificially suppress the production of cholesterol. Now you are leaving the body unprotected. You have switched off the water dousing the fire. Are you aware more people die from low cholesterol than high?

Nature does not produce fevers, colds, inflamed tonsils, diarrhoea and pain just to inconvenience you when are trying to get to work. These are natural and necessary healing reactions. Shouldn't we let them run their course, or listen to what they are telling us, rather than suppress them?

'A 2014 study involving over 60,000 men diagnosed with prostate cancer, found suppressing testosterone levels with drugs was unnecessary and harmful, and did not prolong survival.'

Suppression does not cure disease. It CAUSES it.

The Diagnostic Dance

The average length of time a Doctor spends with you, during an appointment, is 3 minutes. Within 30 seconds he has already made up his mind and stopped listening to you. A remarkable diagnostic feat. If he or she cannot figure out what is wrong, specialists using MRIs, blood tests, x-rays, CT scans, allergy testing, angiograms, colonoscopy, ultrasound and more, can. My local hospital offers 88 different diagnostic tests. Whether they are invasive, harmful, expensive or misleading, does not seem to matter. We undergo these tests even when healthy. An army of 'worried well' attend Well Man and Well Woman clinics, drumming up new business for public and private hospitals. It makes good business sense. Drawn in by my need to know, I paid for a comprehensive 'Well Man' screening at my local private hospital. Test results came back normal, except my total cholesterol was a little high, according to their 'catch-all' low threshold. According to my 'you-aren't-catching-me-with-your-nonsense' threshold, it was fine. Statins were recommended (profits from Statins have been stupendous) which I declined. I have no faith in the High Cholesterol = Heart Disease theory, the test threshold, or the safety of Statins. Alternative medicine is heading the same way, with Applied Kinesiology, Electro acupuncture (VEGA), Darkfield Microscopy, Hair Mineral Analysis and provocation testing, creating opportunities for treatments and the sale of supplements.

There is a risk, in our efforts to understand WHY we are sick, of being led a merry diagnostic dance. Moving from one specialist to another, using different diagnostic tools, checking minor data points, of little real importance, the results of which are invariably inaccurate. The scandalous PSA test, one example. If one test flags a problem, further investigation is needed and off we go for more tests, often invasive and dangerous. Sometimes the practitioner is confident what is wrong, only to have a test contradict him. I was diagnosed by a specialist in one of the top hospitals in the country, with Celiac Disease, only for a confirmation test to come back negative. I could see the specialist's confusion as he suggested more tests. I had seen a dozen other practitioners before him and was getting tired with the expense and constantly changing diagnoses, so thanked him and walked away. It seemed pointless anyway because I already knew, whatever the test result, he was not going to cure me. In his world, auto-immune disorders are 'Incurable'. That confirmation test cost me years looking for other causes. What neither of us knew at the time, was his test was negative because I had not eaten any gluten foods for the few days prior to the test. So no antibodies showed up. Had he asked what I had been eating, I could have told him.

There is a major problem within the U.S. and increasingly, other western nations, of 'over-medicalization'. This has been recognized by the **ABIM**

(**American Board of Internal Medicine**) representing more than 350,000 American doctors. In 2012 it recommended we get less medical care. Their concern? Too many wasteful and unnecessary medical tests, treatments and procedures. In the UK, 1 in 7 operations are deemed unnecessary. I do not think anyone is listening.

Which sadist invented the mammogram? Put your breast in a mangle once a year, irradiate it and this will protect you. Only a man could come up with such a device. What is wrong with breast cancer screening? Well, to start with, up to 30% of lumps in the breast will disappear on their own, without any intervention. Over the last 30 years, it was recently revealed, more than 1 million women were subjected to chemo, radiation and mastectomies, with all the consequences that brings, including death. There was only one problem. They did NOT have breast cancer, after all. Likewise hundreds of thousands of men with prostate cancer.

According to this 2012 review by **The Cochrane Collaboration**

'...for every 2000 women invited for screening throughout 10 years, 1 will avoid dying of breast cancer and 10 healthy women, who would not have been diagnosed if there had not been screening, will be treated unnecessarily. Furthermore, more than 200 women will experience important psychological distress including anxiety and uncertainty for years because of false positive findings.'

'Over-medicalization' is not the only problem with screening mammograms. My conclusion, after reading the latest research (known for decades by the alternative community) is mammograms cause more harm than good.

Testing a few data points, out of thousands of possibilities, is a lucrative business. Tests will increase under the proposed 'Precision Medicine Initiative', which seeks to identify genes which are markers for disease. You identify a gene, which suggests an increased risk of this, or that, disorder. If it is decided you are at risk, drug 'therapy' will almost certainly be prescribed to 'protect' you, while you change your heart-unhealthy or cancer-inducing lifestyle. Since no testing is perfect, there are going to be false positives and false negatives. We know genes can be switched off and on, so this huge backing of genetics seems like just another corporate opportunity to make pots of money, while giving the patient little actual health benefit and a whole heap of additional worry.

"Your test results have come back, Mrs Smith. You have a 55% chance of developing Multiple Sclerosis".

I wonder if Mrs Smith is going to have peace of mind after hearing that? What is clear from this initiative is public health measures targeting the obvious causes of ill health – fake 'food', pollution, lack of exercise, poor parenting, poverty and excess sugar, will be ignored in favor of 'Individualized Medicine'. Corporations will profit from the genetic test, follow-up tests, treatments and an expanded market for every possible disease. No symptoms now but your genes predict trouble ahead. Here's some shiny new pills for 'prevention'. Mrs Smith, of course, even if the test is accurate, is not going to change her ways. If you cannot change people's behavior now, what makes you think you can in the future? I confidently predict there will be no improvement in the nation's health. Pharmaceutical stocks are a BUY.

Alternative tests do not escape criticism. There are a high number of false positives. Many, like muscle-response, or VEGA testing, are dependent on the skill of the operator. If the practitioner gives too much weight to the tests, without confirming via symptoms, we can end up with the wrong treatment for the wrong disorder. In these circumstances, testing is damaging, costing us time, energy and money and arguably our lives, focusing on the wrong problem.

There is a different way to approach our 'Need to Know'. Forget it. Yes, you read correctly. Forget it. Diseases can be resolved without a diagnosis. How? In India, Thailand and Hong Kong, the Ayurvedic, Traditional Chinese Medicine (TCM), Homeopathic and Nature Cure Doctors I met, could not afford expensive gadgets and tests for their patients. They simply got on with the job of creating health, knowing that, if you apply the fundamentals of Natural Healing, illness will resolve. The ancients believed a clean body, provided with proper nutrition, would stay healthy. While a dirty body, lacking nutrients, would sicken and die. There were no such things as clinical trials. They observed nature. We do the same inside our homes. Place a houseplant in good soil, give it clean water and watch it thrive and blossom. Transplant it into poor soil and watch it weaken, fail to bloom and pests and fungi will attack it. Reverse the process and the plant thrives again. The greatest influence on the health of the plant is the quality of the soil. The 'Biological Terrain'.

Where I live in Thailand, animal welfare activists commendably brought an end to dog meat appearing on the nation's menu. Unfortunately, their success had a downside. The number of stray dogs in the country exploded. Dogs are everywhere, emaciated and weak, infested with parasites, their skin scaly, fur dry and patchy, often dying from road accidents, neglect and starvation. If you take them in, deal with the parasites and feed them, their bodies fill out and their fur grows back. Add some tender loving care and they thrive. No chemistry. No pathology. No clinical trials. Just biology and common sense. Biological laws are the same for us as they are for houseplants and stray dogs. When our body's defences are weak, when our 'biological terrain' is poor, we are open to viral, bacterial, fungal and parasitic infection. We can conduct tests to identify which bacteria, viruses or microbes and deal with them but does it really matter we know? Simply clean the body (includes removing parasites) and give it the nutrients needed to strengthen its vitality and defences (immune system) and we get better. This method of healing has operated successfully for thousands of years.

I have witnessed, many times, people recover from illness without knowing precisely what was wrong with them or what exactly cured them. Most traditional healers could not tell you precisely what cured their patients. Natural healing is not the same as symptom-based medicine. If you improve diet, exercise, dissolve emotional stress, take herbs & vitamins, add hydrotherapy, relaxation training, meditation, breathing exercise, acupuncture, a chiropractor and any number of other techniques and your health recovers, how do you know which of these cured you? It is impossible. An herbal combination can include multiple herbs, with many different actions, acting synergistically. According to **Dr Duke's Phytochemical and Ethnobotanical Database**, Mangosteen, a delicious Asian fruit, has 245 distinct actions on the body. How do you know which actions or phytochemicals, within the fruit, triggered healing? You don't. That is just one fruit. Now introduce a half dozen other ingredients AND add all the other healing techniques. This infinite number of variables is the main reason, when you investigate alternative methods of healing, sceptics describe them as "untested"; "unproven"; "no clinical trials" or "not supported by the science". What they don't tell you is it is impossible to prove natural healing works, using current testing paradigms. You are not testing one chemical against one symptom.

"Drugs make a well person sick. How can drugs make a sick person well?"

Abram Hoffer, MD

The Staggering Toll

The U.S. and, increasingly, other industrialized nations, are being overwhelmed by chronic disease. What is a chronic disease? These are ongoing, generally incurable, illnesses or conditions such as heart disease, asthma, cancer and diabetes. Chronic disease is the leading cause of death and disability in the United States. Today, 133 million Americans – 45% of the population – have at least one chronic disease.

Chronic disease is responsible for seven out of every 10 deaths in the U.S. Below are the latest available numbers for the most common chronic disorders.

Allergies	50 million adults suffer nasal allergies. Worldwide, allergies among school children are 40%-50%.
Arthritis	52.5 million (22.7%) of adults.
Asthma	18.9 million (8.2%) adults and 7 million (9.5%) children.
Alzheimer's	231,900 nursing home residents.
Cancer each	230,000 women will get breast cancer this year. The same number of men will get prostate cancer. 2 million new cases year. 1 in 2 men and 1 in 3 women will develop cancer.
Diabetes	30 million. 1.9 million new cases each year. 86 million have pre-diabetes.
Epilepsy	2.8 million cases
Heart Disease	26.5 million. 1 in 6 men and 1 in 10 women will die
COPD	24 million have impaired lung function.
Obesity	70% of adults are overweight or obese
Sinusitis	Affects 13% of adults over 18

Christa

72-year old Christa, from Switzerland, was suffering from too many years of smoking. You could hear her wheezing as she breathed. After two incidents of collapsing, she discovered she was a Type II diabetic. Her A1C reading was 7.8 and fasting blood sugar 177. The normal range is 80-120. Above that and the body starts to suffer damage. Christa was placed on insulin, then Metformin.

Christa's family and friends were understandably concerned about her health. After learning she did not have to suffer this disorder, they encouraged her to sign up for a 21-day 'Reverse Diabetes' program. This involved 10 to 14 days of juice-fasting, followed by 7-11 days of a raw vegan or (LCHF) low carb, high fat diet. In the face of official opinion diabetes is incurable, Christa had her doubts. These were dispelled when Christa's blood sugar readings quickly reverted to normal.

A big concern was whether Christa could kick her long-time smoking habit. This proved to be far easier than she thought, thanks to an herbal tincture which eliminated her tobacco cravings. Stopping proved to be a breeze. Christa came off all her medications and ditched the cigarettes. A heavy coating on her tongue, throughout her 14 days of juice-fasting, showed how 'dirty' or toxic her body was. After 20 years of coughing and wheezing, Christa now breathes easily. Her COPD has resolved. Throughout the program her fasting blood sugars stayed within normal ranges. She also shed some excess pounds. Christa can be pleased with herself. Not least because she is a remarkable lady. Determined, compliant (she stuck to her program), very sociable and easy to look after.

We try not to celebrate too quickly, since the proof of the Retreat pudding lies in the eating. How well people do AFTER the program. Some heal completely within 21 days. Some take longer and need to stay on a low-carb diet for a few more weeks. Some fall back into old patterns, inviting disease to return.

Christa now knows she can maintain improved health, with nutrition. We wish her many more years of life!

Rise of the Health Coach

A million health 'experts' are online. Like town-hall barkers, they vie for our attention and money. The result is confusion. We cannot separate truth from lies, spin from substance. The choices open to us are endless and bewildering. Everything seems to cause everything. Have you noticed? If your disease is not caused by a lack of Vitamin C or D, it is Candida or B12. Echinacea and DX-64 'Bio'-thingamabob can fix it. Purchase this supplement for $24.99 and all will be well. Until you discover there is NO Echinacea in 90% of over-the-counter (OTC) Echinacea products and the herbs you just purchased are so weak you need 20 capsules a day to feel any effect. With practices like this, how can any of us get well? The poor quality of OTC products is one reason I learned how to make my own herbal remedies. (Later, I share the secret).

Surveys tell us 50% of patients, on leaving a Doctor appointment, have no idea what their Doctor just told them. If you are being treated with 'German Biological Medicine', which is highly technical, you can pretty much make it 100%. In the last few years, conventional medicine has acknowledged there is a problem with patients not being able to follow instructions given by their Doctors. The stock advice to change diet, exercise more and reduce stress is not being complied with. How can people be expected to change their unhealthy ways if they do not understand what they are supposed to do and lack quality information and support? They need guidance, encouragement and help, which Doctors do not have the time to provide. Doctors believe 99% of patients who need to change their lifestyle, will fail. With attitudes like that, it is safe to say your Doctor is not going to be of much help.

Clearly we have a problem. Lucky for us, there is a solution. In March 2013 UK Health Minister Anna Soubry urged the **National Health Service** (NHS) in England, and local teams, to take "urgent action" to support Cancer Recovery patients and provide them with a proper Cancer Recovery Plan. The need for support, not only with cancer recovery but other conditions, has given rise to the relatively new profession of 'Health Coach'. In the U.S., Health Coaches, Wellness Coaches, Life and Fitness Coaches are already part of the landscape. A Health Coach bridges the gap between Doctor and patient. It is an excellent idea. In the UK, NHS nurses are being trained for this role. However, it does not bode well. When Cancer wards and hospital food consists of soda and sugary biscuits and nurses are being taught there is no difference between organic and processed food, no amount of 'coaching' is going to restore health. 50% of NHS nurses are obese. These are the people teaching you and I about nutrition!

Health Coaches come in various flavours and with differing levels of expertise and experience. I have adopted the label of Health Coach, since it seems the most appropriate fit. Instead of conventional approaches, I champion Natural and Alternative. Helping those suffering chronic disease like Cancer, Diabetes and Arthritis, to recover from, or better manage, their conditions. An ideal Health Coach has a broad understanding of healing methods, knows what works and what doesn't, what supplements are useful and which are not. They would understand what you should be eating, what will keep you well and provide support as you make needed lifestyle changes. Health Coaches work WITH you, to move you away from building disease, toward building health.

When people come to me, confused and frustrated, I feel compelled to help. If you have knowledge which might help others, how can you not? It was never my intention to travel this path. Friends would mention their health problems and were surprised at my knowledge and pleased when I pointed them toward solutions. They had never heard of Ayurveda or Nature Cure, Ornish or Esselstyn, The Thomsonian School of Healing, Father Kneipp, Benedict Lust, Orthomolecular Medicine and too many others to mention. They thought a body cleanse was a packet of detox tea bags or a Princess Diana colonic.

I taught them Yoga but not like they had been taught before. Advanced breathing exercises they never knew existed. Gave them weight loss and nutritional advice, tapped on their meridians, helped them quit smoking and sobbed with them as traumas were exposed and dissolved. Then they started to ask me to design Detox and Healing programs. To support them as they went through them. To be 'on call' if anything went wrong. To be their Alternative Medicine and Natural Healing 'Guru'. I never imagined I would find myself, today, writing health books, leading Retreats and providing health and wellness guidance over the internet. I prefer a quiet life.

There is another reason I never imagined reaching this point. I should be dead. If I had stayed with conventional medical Doctors and Psychiatrists, I have no doubt I would have committed suicide or been in a wheelchair, crippled with Arthritis, Celiac Disease, Fibromyalgia, chronic depression and debilitating anxiety. Taking painkillers, anti-depressants, beta-blockers, muscle-relaxants, anti-inflammatories and hypoglycaemia meds. Adding $1.5 million dollars to the corporate balance sheet. Instead I Fired My Doctor and Cured Myself.

You can do the same. It's a little scary firing your Doctor. It means flying solo into a world of complexity and competing claims. If you find you are struggling, for whatever reason, seek help. Track down a Naturopath, Health Coach or call some of the other teachers and holistic practitioners out there doing good work. One conversation really could change your life. Try not to be too hard on them, though. After all, we are coming out of a Dark Age of Medicine where, for the last 100+ years, modern medicine has had its own 'Bypass Age'. Where, what could heal you was bypassed in favour of what could be patented, synthesized and monetized. Cures and exciting research laying buried in libraries, suspiciously un-indexed, for 50 years or more, is being unearthed as a wave of practitioners and researchers resurrect the lost Art of Healing.

It is an exciting time but also worrying. The forces of conservatism will not give up passively. They know every trick in the book. After all, they have had a century of practice. You see it with the health supplements Industry. 'Big Pharma' had no need to duke it out with natural supplement companies, who started eating into their market share. It simply bought them up, converted the natural ingredients to synthetic and wrapped them in fancy packaging at hugely inflated prices.

You don't buy a single herb, vitamin or skin cream anymore. Now it's a 'Cellular', 'Nutraceutical', 'Bio-Nano', 'Skin-Whitening', 'Anti-Aging' System, with an air-brushed picture of an impossibly-thin, female model with bleached teeth and a nose-job (in Asia these models look like aliens). You can no longer find skin creams. They are 'serums'. When I see the dazzling cosmetics panels in stores, I shake my head and pass by. The health supplements and cosmetics markets are multi-billion dollar, deceptive-marketing obscenities. I know. I worked in the industry and saw the chemicals used. Some of them so harsh, well-known brands would farm production out to other companies because their workers would get sick. I know how little they cost to make and how much 'natural' product goes into them. The $100 'serum' you just bought? $1 to manufacture.

How can people like me help those who feel overwhelmed and confused? Can't you just go straight to an Ayurvedic Dr., Naturopath or Chiropractor? You can. Just understand alternative practitioners have a right to make a living, have mortgages to pay and families to take care of. Unlike your GP, they spend more than three minutes with you. They are not subsidized by the State and do not get free trips to Disneyland for pushing over-priced meds.

Some alternative practitioners have taken the lead from conventional Doctors. They know you are not going to change your ways, so do what conventional Doctors do. Instead of pharmaceutical medicines, they prescribe herbal remedies and supplements. These will not harm you but, alone, are unlikely to heal you. This is not such a bad thing. If you are not going to change your lifestyle, at least bolster your defences. Herbs can be protective. I call them my 'clean-up' crew. For instance, Milk Thistle protects the liver, when you are still drinking. Hawthorn Berry, the heart. Fresh, raw garlic, high blood pressure and certain cancers. Bitter herbs, diabetes. They will not harm you in the same way pharmaceuticals do. Just make sure there is some actual herb in the bottle and not a weak decoction of leftover twigs, sprayed with pesticides, shipped over, irradiated and gassed, from somewhere in the third world.

The quality of herbal supplements is a major issue. In February 2015, the **New York Attorney General**'s Office asked major retailers Wal-Mart, Walgreens,

Target and GNC, to halt sales of certain herbal supplements. 79% of their herbal supplements were found to have NO herbal DNA. The worst offender was Wal-Mart, with 96% of their supplements having no DNA from plants listed on their labels.

Tens of millions today are suffering chronic degenerative disorders. The only chance they have of reversing their disorders is to change their disease-inducing ways. To detoxify all the poisons and pollutants, improve their diet, reduce stress and get their bodies moving. Changing lifestyle is, literally, a life or death decision. It sounds simple when you see it written down but like New Year Resolutions, which last all of 5 minutes, it is not easy to make lasting changes. Knowledgeable patients understand they cannot get well without guidance and support. An army of health tourists regularly descend upon Detox Retreats and Spas in Thailand, Malaysia, Mexico and elsewhere, to enjoy Wellness and Healing programs. Why? Because they know if they undertake programs at home, without support, they will fail. There are too many temptations, distractions and resistance from others. They may also lack the necessary knowledge. In an holistic retreat setting - it does not matter if it is a white-glove, five-star spa or a simple hut on the beach - the support, education and attention they receive is fundamental to kick-starting lifestyle changes. Many times I hear those enjoying Retreats say, "This is the best thing I ever did for myself".

Not everyone can afford to jet off to sunny climes. This is where the Internet becomes a saviour. Imagine being able to consult face-to-face with a Health or Wellness Coach over the Internet, using online video software like 'Skype', from the comfort and privacy of your living room or office? Skype calls are free. It certainly beats trudging to the Doctor's surgery, waiting in line on a cold winter's day, for 3 minutes of attention, then walking out mystified by what you were just told, clutching a bag full of side effects. Accessing the Coach's online calendar allows you to select your preferred time. What kinds of questions do people ask a Health Coach? They range from the basic:

"How do I detox my kids from Fluoride?"

To the serious:

"The Doctor has put me on Warfarin. Is there an herbal equivalent?

"I want to try juice-fasting but it is too cold to drink raw juices. What can I do?

Pleas for help:

"My husband says alternative medicine is 'mumbo-jumbo' and is being difficult. Can you talk to him?"

Wailing and gnashing of teeth:

"I am tired of this diet. Can I have a glass of wine and a steak, PLEASE!" (They know the answer but I do commend them for trying).

Panic:

"I started my detox and woke up feeling awful. Should I stop?"

"Help! I'm trying to come off anti-depressants and feel overwhelmed with anxiety and suicidal thoughts!" (Not funny. I have been through it).

Then the good stuff which makes it all worthwhile...

"It's unbelievable. My depression has lifted!"

"I feel amazing!"

"All my symptoms have gone!"

"Thank you. You saved me a fortune".

"I had no idea it was so easy!"

Finally, from a friend with diabetes:

"I can see!"

No. I don't cure the blind, nor do I raise the dead. He meant he could see better.

If this sounds a little like blowing my own trumpet, of course I am, but there is a serious purpose in sharing such examples with you. People are lost, even though they have access to incredible amounts of information and no shortage of experts. It is hardly surprising. The experts don't agree with each other. No sooner have they made one discovery, a few years later, they overturn it with another. No apology or mea culpa. They simply present the new diet or 'revolution', in a flurry of publicity, without missing a beat.

There is so much to know. So many options available. Just look at diets. Where do you even start? There have been thousands of different diets foisted on the public over the last 100 years. Yet, NOT knowing what to eat can be costly. If my Naturopathic friend is correct, I could have been cured in 3 days. Instead, it took 20 years. In that period my efforts to recover my health, loss of job and expected future earnings, cost me around £600,000. If I include future income from raises, bonuses and promotions, it could easily be £1 million. I was an Information Technology (I.T.) expert.

I cannot speak for you, since your circumstances will be different but if I had encountered someone who understood the different methods of healing... Modern, Complementary, Alternative and Natural... when I first began to struggle, I might have been spared my long ordeal. Do I believe there is benefit in paying for a Health Coach? It depends who it is. There are good and bad in all professions, but if I had my time over again, I would be on the phone in a heartbeat. Experience is a great teacher.

Who might benefit from talking to a Health Coach? Those:

- Seeking clarity
- Lacking a healing program or struggling to understand one
- Needing guidance, support and inspiration
- 'Grasshoppers', who hop from therapy to therapy
- Checking they are being given good advice

At Antarana we never know who is going to walk through our doors and with what set of conditions. It is fascinating how unique is an individual's history, character, personality traits, habits, hopes and fears. They need individualized, customized solutions. Not standardized, complex specializations no-one can understand.

One of our biggest health challenges is taking what we learn and applying it. We are not all motivated, or learn, the same way. Some can be sat with a book open in front of them and an instructional video playing, yet still not understand. These types need to be taken by the hand and shown. Stress can play a role. Stress blocks our ability to take in new information, comprehend what we are seeing, or take action.

Others who come unstuck are the knowledgeable, who have no practical experience. Their knowledge, even if extensive, remains at the level of the intellect. Some of the prominent speakers I see would not be able to handle bowel cleanses or cope with someone who needs emotional healing. They connect easily with a large audience but struggle one-on-one with someone in crisis. The best practitioners are those who have been through the school of hard knocks and are not simply armed with book-knowledge. The best person to counsel a recovering alcoholic is a recovered alcoholic. The best person to cleanse your body is someone who has conducted cleanses (detox). The best person to take you through a healing program is someone who has healed others and themselves.

Theoretical knowledge is fine but how do you, step-by-step, conduct your program and see it through to completion?

- Do you know what a 'healing crisis' is and how to respond to it?
- If you are conducting a deep cleanse of the body, how do you know when the body is clean?

- What if you cannot find quality foods or supplements?

- Should you keep taking the medication the Doctor has prescribed?

- What happens if the herbal remedies/vitamins/juices aren't working?

Many questions can arise.

When you purchase a house or business, you will often hear the most important three factors are 'Location, Location, Location.' In health, it is 'Education, Education and Education.' Educating retreat guests and Skype callers takes up much of my time. Whether it is teaching nutrition, explaining natural methods of healing or recommending which (not 'Witch') Doctor to use. People need help navigating it all.

Over the years I wasted thousands of pounds on tests and treatments which failed to properly diagnose my condition or its cause. Few would have been necessary had I been better informed or had someone independent to ask. Today, with years of research and practical experience behind me, I know pretty much what works and what doesn't. Where I do not know, I know where to look, or will turn to colleagues such as Paul Johnson, MD., a former Paediatrician and Oxford researcher who, even as I type, is using science to prove the value of ancient breathing techniques in balancing the nervous system. His vast experience and no-nonsense, academic mind can sniff out a bogus therapy in a heartbeat.

Nobody Cures You

No Doctor Cures You

No Alternative Practitioner Cures You

No Natural Healer Cures You

One of the greatest errors in medicine is the belief someone else cures us. I need to make it clear and you need to understand, nobody is going to stand over you with a magic wand and say, "Abracadabra! You are healed."

The great natural healing systems of the world all understand THE BODY CURES ITSELF. Which is why the title of the book is 'Fire Your Doctor Cure Yourself' The goal of all practitioners should be to fire up and support the body's own self-healing mechanism, remove all impediments to healing and provide it with the materials it needs to repair itself. The body then heals. And when it heals, it does not just heal your Cancer, Heart Disease, Diabetes or Arthritis. It heals all of them. As Charlotte Gerson says, "You cannot heal one disease and keep two others. When one heals, they all heal". The focus of natural healing is not so much the disease itself (the name we give is not so important) but cleaning and strengthening the body. If you are fortunate and have a Naturopath near you, you may wish to enlist their help. Many people are not fortunate. They lack the finances to pay practitioner fees and for healthier diets or supplements. Cancer bankrupts many, who not only have to absorb the cost of conventional treatment but the cost of recovery, which can also be significant.

All is not lost. You can still do some things, such as Yoga, which is free and needs little space or equipment. Or simple stretches and exercises. Fasting and Water Cures (I talk about these later) cost pennies. The ancients did not drive BMWs or have the latest iPhone. In some societies there was no such thing as money, or 'medicine', or even a medical profession. Yet people still healed.

No matter one's budget, if you are suffering a chronic, degenerative disorder (or wish to avoid one) you are going to have to take matters into your own hands, accept responsibility for your disease and do something you have not tried before. Instead of building disease, build health. Instead of relying on others, rely on yourself. It is amazing what the body can do, if given a chance. Miracles can happen if you believe in yourself and take responsibility for your own well-being. The good news is, for most disorders, healing can happen quickly. The great natural healers will tell you, they see patients who had been sick for decades, throw off their disease in a matter of days. I see it myself, when counselling. With EFT and our 'Breaking The Chains' technique; traumas, or addictions, which have been tormenting people for years, dissolve in minutes.

How is this possible? I could try to impress you with some pseudo-scientific explanation of how these techniques work but often it is simply the first time people have seriously attempted to address the problem. They did not know they could.

In these pages I present a healing program that draws on the simplest (in my experience) techniques from both the ancient and modern healing systems of the world. A program that can be conducted at a Retreat, a cabin in the woods or in your own home. You can even choose the pace at which you wish to recover. If you are frail, take it slowly. It may take 18 months. If stronger, 6 months. If you are prepared to put in a sustained effort, 30 days or less. It would be wrong of me to claim every disorder is healed, every time. We are all different. However, once you read and understand how the method works, you will see it has the potential to do what it says on the tin. One key to healing is not whether a method is unique (there are many roads to Rome) but how diligently you apply it.

If you are someone who believes your disease or disorder is 'incurable' because that's what the Doctor told you, rid yourself of the idea right now. I personally do not believe Mother Nature (or whatever name you use) is so cruel she would deny anyone the ability to heal. By the way. It is not going to be as before, with a Doctor dispensing a few pills. Healing is going to require your full participation.

YOU decide whether you will act and see it through to completion. YOU decide to stop doing whatever you are doing that is making you sick. YOU decide what you put in your mouth. YOU decide whether to move your body, or flop on the couch, spellbound by a TV, computer or smartphone. YOU decide whether to feed your mind useful, useless, negative or positive thoughts.

Of one thing you can be sure. If you do nothing, you will stay sick. Nobody is going to come along and sprinkle you with pixie-dust. If you are only prepared to give healing two days of effort, this book is not for you.

"In the history of humanity there has never been a disease that someone, somehow, somewhere has not eradicated, removed the disease from their body and totally healed. Can what they did work for you? Is there a reason why it should not?"

Sharon Forrest

100 Doctors

Once Upon a Time there was a powerful King who had 100 doctors looking after his health. The finest Doctors in the land. Soon, one of the older Doctors passed away and a search began for a replacement. Many candidates came to be interviewed. Each candidate had to correctly answer one question from each of the other 99 Doctors. All failed. One day a candidate arrived who answered all the questions correctly. The King congratulated him and welcomed him as the 100th Doctor. The Doctor said,

"Your Highness. I would like to ask the other ninety-nine Doctors a question".

The King, intrigued, agreed.

"What are the two most important things for health?"

All of the Doctors answered. None correctly.

"What are they?" asked the King, intensely curious.

"A walk in the morning and an hour in the sunshine" he replied.

So pleased was the King with this answer, he fired all the other 99 Doctors. The new Doctor became the most famous physician of his Age.

This ancient story is a reminder of how, in a world filled with complex remedies and impenetrable jargon, preventing illness and maintaining our health can be quite simple. The two most important things for health have, arguably, not changed.

Exercise

How many of you take a walk in the morning and enjoy an hour in the sunshine? When I was in the military, exercise would commence at first light. In the Mediterranean, walking is common, particularly after a meal. There is something magical about the cool early morning air. While the rest of the country is sleeping, an early morning walk is invigorating and ensures greater mental sharpness for the rest of the day. Exercise during the day helps you sleep better at night. It also helps with constipation, reduces the risk of breast and colon cancer, burns calories and gets more oxygen into body and brain. Getting our circulation moving improves sexual health, muscles get stronger and so do the bones of osteoporosis patients. Immune function strengthens, 'bad' cholesterol drops, stress reduces and physical tension is released. Walking briskly each day can reduce your risk of heart disease by 40%.

A morning walk is not so easy when you work shifts, live in a city, do not feel safe outside or only have time for a mad dash to work. Here you must do what you can. Exercise later in the day. If you cannot walk, get on your bike. If you cannot do that, learn some simple breathing and stretching exercises. One fun exercise I do each morning is a Qigong exercise called 'Tossing the Ball'. It is perfect for almost everyone, including the overweight and less mobile. It can also be used to dissolve toxic emotions. Instead of 'tossing' a ball, imagine you are tossing away anger, fear, hatred, heartbreak or frustration. This exercise can be conducted slowly, or at an increased pace, becoming a super workout. It does not need any equipment, costs nothing and you don't have to move from one spot. You can search for it online or watch for a video on the Antarana website.

There is a problem with government guidelines on exercise. The same problem we find with taking medicines, or with the food we eat. We aren't all the same! 20% of people, doing the typical exercise we see in gyms, do not see the benefits they are seeking or expecting. These are called 'non-responders', while 15% do exceptionally well and are called 'super-responders'. The type of exercise chosen needs to be tailored to individual need and response. You may have heard of Personalized Medicine? Welcome to Personalized Exercise. Genetic tests claim to be able to identify what most of us can observe. If you are a 'non', 'low' or 'super' responder. These tests also suggest an exercise plan (for a few dollars more) but many test only one single data point and are unreliable. Buyer beware.

My own reluctance to flogging myself in a gym, is a lack of interest in being in the same company as steroid-munching gorillas, preening hedonists and those using it as a pick-up joint. I will always be more Mr Bean than Arnold Schwarzenegger. Whatever the claims of genetic testing, it was my observation that, no matter the body type, or response, a two week Royal Marine training course leaves everyone bursting with energy. The military have taken millions through rigorous training, over a hundred years, so you would think they would know all about responders or non-responders. Yet, when I served, I never heard of this. I could see some of my colleagues were natural marathon runners (endurance) and some short distance sprinters (speed) but all undertook the same exercise and all benefited. Yes, military strength, fitness and endurance training are hard core. Hardly suited to the over 50s, with arthritic knees, carrying too much weight. They need gentle, introductory, strength-building programs to get tendons and ligaments ready for more vigorous exercise. Otherwise, injury rates are high. Message being... Don't run before you can walk!

The obvious danger of a genetic test reporting you as a 'non-responder' is it provides you with the perfect excuse to do nothing. Does "It's genetic" sound familiar? You won't see any value in exercise at all. Don't buy into this. There are numerous health benefits to moving the body, not just weight loss or muscle gain.

Sunshine

What about the sun? We have been taught to fear it. Why? Vitamin D is crucial for protecting us against Cancer, and sunshine on our skin produces it. Sunshine is an anti-depressant. Don't we feel miserable in the darker months in the northern hemisphere? Except for a few rare instances, most of us need MORE sunshine, not less. Heliotherapy (sun-bathing) is an important part of 'Nature Cure' and included in our programs. There is no need for us to be fearful of the sun just because some industry 'expert' says it is bad for us (wants to sell more sunscreen), and a few have overdone it. Everything in moderation. Go out in the sun when it is not too high in the sky. Make sure you do not burn. Too much sun, like too much of anything, is bad for you. But so is too little.

Christians and Yoga

Christianity in the U.S. has a large following while, in the UK, it is very much on life support with less than 4% of the population actively practicing. Christians sometimes worry about Eastern disciplines, like Yoga, concerned they are gateways to worshipping 'false gods' or distractions from living a purely Christian life. Are these concerns justified?

Were you aware Dr Dean Ornish' Heart Program, which reverses heart disease using diet, exercise and stress reduction, was given to him by a Hindu Swami? Knowing this, would you reject it? Is a Hindu REALLY worshipping a 'false' god? Or is he perhaps worshipping the many faces of ONE god? The same God you worship?

Many years ago, when dipping a toe in the spiritual waters, I asked a priest if Christianity had an exercise program? I had begun to practice yoga. He replied, "Stay away from Yoga. It is used by Satan to seduce Christians away from their faith." This sounded rather dramatic and unlikely. If one's Christian faith is so weak one can be seduced by a towel and exercise mat, perhaps the problem isn't so much Yoga but one's own lack of faith.

The 'New Age' movement encourages spiritual seekers to experiment with astrology, astral projection, crystals, Ouija boards, Tarot, mediums and so on. This certainly is a cause for concern. One might wonder what is so wrong with traditional Christianity people are rejecting it in favour of alternatives? It is an unfortunate reality any mention of 'Christianity' or 'God', to those who come to see me, will cause their eyes to glaze over and they will be out of the door, like a greyhound after a rabbit. In their view, organized religion is discredited and degraded. Hardly surprising when you are constantly assailed by stories of priestly paedophiles and religions at war. Please don't get me started on Televangelists. You don't need to see a trident and horns to know the 'devil' is at work with these money-grubbing 'false prophets'.

Christian web sites warn a popular greeting, 'Namaste', means 'I bow to the god within you.' A billion people on this earth greet each other by clasping their hands together and bowing in respect. Including millions of Christians in India. Should a western Christian cause offense and run away, so they are not seen to be 'bowing to another god?' Or simply be courteous and return the greeting? After all, if there IS only one God, how could there be another 'god' within them? I like the Asian way of greeting. It is more sanitary than shaking unclean hands and better than wincing from some smirking brute with a handshake which can crush stone.

'Om' is a Sanskrit word, associated with Yoga, which alarms some Christians. This is odd, since 'Om' is in reality spelled A-U-M. 'Aum', 'Amen'. 'Aum', 'Amen'. See the similarity? They have the same linguistic root.

I have been practicing and teaching Yoga, off and on, for 25 years. Inspired by the man most responsible for the resurgence of modern Yoga in the west, Krishnamacharya. He did not deny the West the benefits of yoga because 'Christians only believe in one God'. Had he done so, we may never have learned of this phenomenal practice. His attitude toward religions and Yoga was only, "That we acknowledge a power greater than ourselves." The religious aspect of Hinduism can be off-putting. His son, Desikachar, studied under him for 28 years, with one condition. No God. Trained as an engineer, he did not want the associated Hindu religious trappings. We see, today, many Yoga disciplines have stripped religion from the practice. Christians can relax. Better still, they can use the opportunity to turn Yoga into 'Christian Yoga'. How so? By injecting their own beliefs into their practice. How might this work? When meditating, replace your mantra with 'Amen'. When doing the 'Sun Salute', imagine you are saluting God or Jesus. If a pose or breathing exercise results in the resolution of a physical ailment, or release of an emotional wound, give thanks to God. What matters is your INTENTION.

There are many styles of Yoga. I cut my teeth on Sivananada Yoga before putting together my own program, tailored to my Constitutional Type and particular needs. I sometimes draw on Iyengar Yoga, which has exercises to treat, or prevent, a wide range of illnesses. The style of Yoga I teach is better described as 'Yoga Therapy'. It is gentle for a reason. Too many people get injured attempting postures their bodies are not ready for. Yoga is a fantastic system which, practiced correctly and safely, brings tremendous health benefits.

There is an aspect of Yoga which falls into the category of 'Spiritual journey'. I would describe myself as a 'Lost Soul' or 'Prodigal Son' who, dissatisfied with life, spent years shopping at the Alternative Healing and Spiritual bazaars. Along the way I encountered many other prodigal sons and lost souls, seeking an alternative to the godless, material, selfish, uncaring world the merchant class has created for us. The class which seeks to destroy God because he is 'competition'. The class that has no problem with religion, provided you worship Pepsi, Nike, Exxon or Apple.

Yoga led me back to Christianity by helping me understand my own religion better. It led me back to Christianity because I recognized it would take me, perhaps, 40 years of Yoga and meditation to achieve what Christian Saints could achieve, overnight, through the power of Grace.

There are some Yoga practices which lead to transcendent states but very few adherents can achieve them. I see the western 'pony-tail and flip-flop brigade' (no offence intended) as seekers. Eventually their seeking will draw them back home. Do not fear them or fear for them. Work on yourself instead. Christians are instructed to 'Let your light so shine you honour your father in heaven'. Instead of worrying about other religions, work on shining your own light, so it attracts others to you. Like a moth to a flame.

Greg

Greg was a typical ex-seaman. 70 years old when he had his third heart attack. A seemingly hopeless case, Greg was grossly overweight, smoked, took no exercise, ate meat-pies and chips and loved his sugary mug of tea. He was on assorted heart medications, beta-blockers, statins, etc., convinced they gave him protection. After his third heart attack, Greg finally got the message. If he didn't change his ways, a fourth would be his last.

I saw Greg 7 months later and was shocked by the difference in him. He had lost 25kg (50lbs) and looked vital and alive. Gone was the walking dead man I knew. Greg told me all his blood work was normal, he had stopped his medication and the Doctor said he was out of danger, as far as his heart was concerned. All this was incredibly good news. I wanted to know the secret to this amazing turnaround. Greg told me he could not completely change his lifestyle. Cycling seemed less arduous than pounding the streets, so he purchased a bicycle. What started out as ½ a mile per day, eventually turned into 15. The change in him, from exercise alone, was impressive.

I would like to say Greg lived happily ever after. Not so. 12 months on, Greg's heart gave out. What Greg had not revealed to me, or his Doctor, was he was still smoking.

I mention this story because it is instructive. People commence their healing programs, begin to feel better, then stop. Before long they have returned to some, or all, of their unhealthy ways. The next thing you hear is they are dead. This is committing suicide with half measures. The lesson? When you start a task, finish it! If Greg had given up smoking he might still be around, his arteries fully restored, living into his 80's or 90's.

David

At 65, David had peripheral arterial disease. The circulation to his legs was increasingly restricted, with smoking the prime culprit. David's lower legs were dark mottled red, his feet almost black. Dramatic action was called for. Surprising everyone, David embarked on a 10-day juice fast at our 'Homestay' Retreat. He stopped smoking and each day had 3 sessions of contrast bathing (hydrotherapy) on his legs and feet, juice-fasting, dry skin brushing, sesame oil massage, swimming and walking. When he left you could definitely see an improvement. How much of an improvement became clear, when a few days after finishing his program, David called to say he had just completed an 8km morning walk on the beach. I am used to seeing dramatic improvement but David's progress was astonishing.

David was understandably delighted and promised to continue the good work after he left the retreat. He would call me every day to say how well he was doing, then suddenly the calls stopped. A wee small voice in my mind said, "He's back drinking again". Sure enough, two weeks later, while dropping my adoptive daughter off at school, I spotted him smoking in the street. My heart sank. "Why, why, why?!" Why would anyone do this after making such brilliant progress? Of course, I knew the answer. David was bored. He lived alone and old habits die hard. It did not take him long to get back to his cigarettes, pals and beer. I am sure he convinced himself he would be okay and told me he still swam regularly. Two years later David died in hospital intensive care, with half his oesophagus removed, his blackened legs scheduled for amputation and his family £25,000 poorer from hospital bills.

One Law people need to understand. Your body does not care for your justifications or delusions. It only experience consequences.

"The art of medicine consists in amusing the patient while nature cures the disease."

Voltaire

Nutrition and Healing

Every cell in our body is created from the food we eat, the water we drink and the air we breathe. The food choices we make influence our mood, energy, appearance, health and wellbeing. Cultures around the world understand this. Hippocrates understood. The great healers understood. We, too, need to understand,

'WE ARE WHAT WE EAT'.

That being so, how is it multinational fast food chains like McDonald's and Burger King are permitted to open outlets in top hospitals, including children's hospitals, selling burgers, nuggets and fries? In March 2015, a UK Parliamentary Committee Report quoted Prof Theresa Marteau, an expert in public health at Cambridge University, who said:

"...it is at best anomalous and at worst negligent that NHS properties continue to serve foods high in sugar, fat and salt, as exemplified by McDonald's and Burger King outlets in some of our most prestigious hospitals, including Guy's hospital in London and Addenbrooke's hospital in Cambridge."

A British cardiologist was less diplomatic...

"It is nothing short of obscene that the very institutions that are supposed to be setting an example of good health, our hospitals, have become a branding opportunity for the junk food industry."

"It is perhaps not surprising that 50% of the NHS 1.4 million employees are themselves overweight or obese. Banning the sale of junk food in hospitals is long overdue."

In Australia, The Royal Children's Hospital in Melbourne has a McDonald's operating inside its building. In the U.S. Chick-fil-A has at least 20 hospital locations, McDonald's at least 18, and Wendy's at least five, according to the Physicians Committee for Responsible Medicine. McDonald's delivers meals right to sick patients' beds. (I wonder if that includes the Heart Ward?) Hospital food is notoriously poor. You can understand why patients and visitors do not wish to eat it. Elderly patients come out of hospitals more malnourished than when they went in. The rate of malnutrition in hospitals today is around 40%.

Many fascinating books and articles have been written about food. The importance of fibre, herbs, vitamins, antioxidants, phytochemicals, enzymes and which diet is best for this or that condition? A great book of this type is 'The Rainbow Diet' by Chris Woollams, who created the CancerActive charity and web site, after his daughter died of a brain tumour. Written to help beat Cancer it is a 'must read' no matter what disorder you have. Not all books are as well written and researched. Many are written by people who have never healed a patient or tossed a Mediterranean salad. They list what herbs are good for cholesterol or constipation and enthuse about 'Superfoods' and raw food diets. This is fine. Proper nutrition is crucial to health. If you can find untainted food, master the recipes and have the motivation to alter and stick with your diet, there is every chance you will see an improvement in your condition. Even a cure.

A focus on nutrition alone can fail because we are more than just the physical body. We are also Emotional, Psychological, Energetic and Spiritual beings. Affected by our outer, as well as inner, environment. We can eat the best food on the planet and the most potent herbs but if their healing factors cannot get to where they are needed, we will see little benefit. If we eat when emotionally upset, indigestion often results, or our food becomes toxic. Even when we decide to change our ways and eat healthily, a cure eludes us because our bodies are loaded with toxins, which need to be eliminated. As Cancer champion Charlotte Gerson informs us...

"You cannot heal a toxic body".

Hippocrates, the 'Father of Modern Medicine', said "Let Food Be Thy Medicine"' but he did not live in a time of 'Agri-business' where genetically-modified 'Frankenfood' was grown in soil stripped of vital nutrients and doused with millions of tons of hazardous chemicals... herbicides, pesticides, fungicides and 'fertilizers'... turning vast tracts of once-fertile, arable land into mineral-deficient, contaminated deserts. He did not live in a time when 70% of the population were obese, their bodies and minds devastated by industrialized oils, fake sugars, msg, trans-fats, preservatives, household cleaning products, insecticides and cosmetics. Seduced into consuming poisons by deceitful marketing, where 'Diet' and 'Low-Fat' make you sick and obese. He did not live in a time when millions of stressed adults and over-stimulated children were turned into 'Zombies' by psychiatrists dispensing 'chemical coshes'.

It is difficult staying healthy or healing a disorder, with a vegetarian diet, if the commercial vegetables you eat are contaminated and deficient in nutrients. Or a vegan diet, if it is unsuitable for your Constitutional or Metabolic Type. You will not thrive and may make yourself sicker. I know. It happened to me.

In today's world, Hippocrates instruction is more important than ever. Only, we need to be more educated in how we approach nutrition. Accordingly, let us take a look at where most of us obtain our nutrition.

There is No Food in a Supermarket

"Everyone else is eating it, so it must be okay"

"Food companies wouldn't harm us. There are laws against it"

"Regulatory bodies protect consumers. It's all tested"

"I am not sick and have been eating this food for years"

"There's no other choice in my area"

"It's cheap, convenient, my favourite foods are all in one place. Why worry?"

What a glittering display lines our supermarket shelves. In the largest stores, you can find 50,000 different products. The choice seems incredible. Most of us shop at the Supermarket or Hyper Market or the local Family Mart. I go regularly. Not to purchase food but to while away an hour or two, indulging in my favourite pastime, 'people-watching'. My trips are both comedy and tragedy. Comedy, because I sometimes spot friends, or those who have been to see me, for advice, racing away from me, with half-filled shopping trolleys. Tragedy, because they don't want me to see the 'treats' filling the trolleys. It's no contest. I am built for speed and invariably catch them. Not to wag a disapproving finger but to reassure them it is okay and not to be embarrassed. Rome isn't built in a day and unless you are highly motivated, you cannot switch from an unhealthy lifestyle, to a healthy one, overnight. You will find it too stressful and give up.

I am different to my friends. Where they see 'food', I see genetically-modified corn, grown in nutritionally-deficient soil, coated in dangerous chemicals, heated, irradiated, re-formed from homogenized gloop into different shapes, mixed with fillers, with added fructose corn syrup (or aspartame), flavourings, colourings, preservatives and any number, from a thousand different chemicals. By the time it emerges from being processed, it has been stripped of live enzymes, natural vitamins and minerals. Some are added back. Only, instead of natural, bio-available nutrients, they use synthetic chemicals and crushed rocks. Put a picture of alien robots or dancing fruit on the box, complete the illusion it is 'food' by printing '100% Natural' and 'Fortified with Vitamins and Minerals!' and watch it fly off the shelf. We give this to our children, when we wouldn't give it to our pets.

Animals aren't confused. They know the garbage we are buying is not food. It may look like food, taste like food, smell like food and they call it food but 'Fido' wouldn't touch it if he was starving. We even tell our children, when they are eating their chips or sodas…"Don't give that to the dog, it's bad for them" without a thought it must also be bad for us. Insanity! It is not just insane. When we feed our children foods lacking in nutrients, saturated with sugar, salt and trans-fats, loaded with calories and laced with chemicals, and they subsequently suffer cancer, diabetes, obesity and so on, what do we call this? Child abuse? Neglect? Manslaughter? You do not want to hear this because you love your children but if you understand the relationship between diet and sickness yet still give your children these foods, what else do you call it?

Why do we do this to our children and to ourselves? It is as if the mind is splintered into separate compartments. One compartment is instinctive. Like the dog, it says, 'stay away from this food'. Another compartment is rational, it knows the food is fattening and toxic and it, too, says, 'stay away from this food'. Another compartment is impressionable. This is the compartment the food companies fill with repetitive, comforting, emotional messages which say 'Drink me. I will make your bones strong'. 'Eat me. I am natural and healthy'. Children's cereals are a good example of this. Looking at one cereal packet recently, I saw the following 'hooks' on the front:

'Simply Nutritious'

'Gluten-Free!'

'No Artificial Colours or Flavours'

'With Whole Grain!'

Encouraging messages, indeed. But hold on a minute. A few are missing:

'High in Poisonous Sugars'

'With added GM FrankenCorn'

'Homogenized and Plasticized'

'Fortified With BHT'

'BHT' is a chemical called Butylated Hydroxytoluene, an endocrine disruptor, linked to cancer in animal studies and banned in Europe. There are far safer additives which do the same job as BHT, yet Food Giants in the U.S. still use it. With selective messages like this and no mention of the down-side, we are seduced into eating it and then guaranteed to keep doing so. These foods have been designed to hook you like a junkie. Food and chemicals are formulated to stimulate your 'Bliss Point'. This is the exact amount of sugar, salt, fat, etc... required to delight the pleasure sensors in your brain. Your resistance weakens and you easily surrender until, months or years later, chronic sickness and/or obesity forces you to wake up from the trance into which you have been placed.

Raw Material

A typical Supermarket meat counter is filled with choice cuts and plump, succulent joints of beef, chicken and pork. How this meat got there is something consumers do not wish think about. Cows, whose evolutionary food is grass, are fed corn, chicken manure or ground-up other cows (known as rendering). 'Mad Cow' disease (BSE) was almost certainly caused by food scientists turning cows into carnivores. Unlike Hollywood depictions of cute talking farm animals, they weren't fed grass but their own chums. Animals are injected with bio-engineered growth hormone, antibiotics, water, glucose, stabilizer and preservatives. Beef doesn't seem quite so succulent when you look at it a little closer. Even less so, when you learn how badly animals are treated. Sadistic violence and abuse by workers toward factory-farmed animals is rampant.

50 billion chickens are raised for meat and eggs worldwide. For years we have considered chicken the lean, healthy choice. Yet the average fat content of supermarket chickens is 17%. So much for 'low-fat'. These poor birds are confined in a tiny space and engineered to grow so quickly their legs are not strong enough to carry them. When legs break, birds die slowly because they cannot reach food or water, or are trampled to death by other birds. Battery hens never get the chance to see the light of day or feel the grass beneath their feet.

Some consumers, disturbed by factory-farming, have turned toward other sources of meat, unaware similar conditions prevail. Egg-laying hens and roosters, used for breeding, are de-beaked between the ages of one-day and five months. This is to prevent feather-pecking other birds. Likewise, turkeys, pheasant, quail, and guinea fowl. Ducks, too, have their bills removed. "Free-range" chickens and turkeys experience the same barbaric treatment. The inhumane conditions cows, chickens, ducks and pigs suffer is a monstrous crime committed by corporate capitalism. A powerful corporate executive, in an office far removed from farm animals, with a remit to drive down costs and increase profits, has no consideration of animal welfare. To him, or her, animals are no more than an entry in a balance sheet. 'Raw material' for the food processing industry.

Got Milk?

For thousands of years mankind has consumed cow's milk. In India, raw milk is used in traditional medicine for healing. Amish people in northern Indiana, drink raw milk. European Union regulations state all raw milk products are legal and considered safe for human consumption. Humans were drinking raw milk, long before Louis Pasteur and his 'Germ Theory' came along. Is raw milk dangerous? From 1998-2008, in the U.S., there were no recorded deaths from drinking raw milk. This cuts no ice with governments who have banned its sale on public health grounds. A curious stance when alcohol and cigarettes kill many, yet are permitted.

Processed milk is not the same as raw milk. Homogenization alters milk's chemistry, while pasteurization destroys nutrients. Processed milk contains traces of hormones, antibiotics, pesticides and faeces. We are encouraged to drink milk by myths like 'calcium is good for the bones', even though four worldwide epidemiological surveys show nations which consume the most calcium have the highest rates of hip fracture. The cause of osteoporosis is not insufficient calcium but a too-acid diet. All animal products are acid-forming in the body. That acidity has to be neutralized. Unless we balance this, with alkaline foods, the body takes calcium from our bones. The irony is the milk and dairy you believe are adding calcium are, in reality, depleting it.

Another bastardization of milk is the addition of sugar. I tasted some store-bought milk recently and spat it out. It was barely recognizable from the milk I drank as a youngster. A pint of 'Gold Top' from the milkman had two inches of cream on the top. What happened to the cream?

In Asia, Africa and many other parts of the world, they do not consume dairy products. It is not a natural part of their diet. However, the height westerners reach encourages parents and governments to give milk to children. In Asia we must seem like giants. I am 6' and am amazed at how many westerners are taller than me. Look at the Dutch, or should that be look UP at the Dutch? In the last 150 years, the average height of Dutch men has increased by 8". In the U.S. it is 2.7". What is making the Dutch grow so rapidly? Their diet is rich in meat and dairy. Could Monsanto's growth hormone rBGH be to blame? Milk is designed to turn a 60lb calf into a 2000lb cow. The calf stops drinking its mother's milk between the ages of 6 to eight months. Yet we 'intelligent' humans are drinking this milk, throughout our lives. Just because we are able to drink it, does not mean we are meant to. No other species continues to drink milk beyond weaning, which should tell us how unnatural it is.

The Illusion of Choice

When you look down the dazzling aisles in a supermarket, you can't fail to be impressed. 30 different cereals, 20 different dog foods. 25 different cans of beans. 40 different detergents. Many different brand names. Yet, what seems to be impressive consumer choice is really just an illusion. Why? Because 6 food giants own almost all of the brands. Many brands are made in the same factory. This is true, also, for organic brands, which we think are independent but have been bought up by the large food conglomerates, unbeknown to the consumer.

Choice? Those 30 different cereals, you see, are made with just three genetically-modified crops. Corn, wheat and oats.

What about supermarket fruits and vegetables? Monoculture farming gives us two varieties of apples, one variety of potato, one variety of carrots. Uniform, bland, tasteless and genetically-modified. Not much consumer choice there. No need to concern yourself with seasons. Fruit and vegetables are available year-round, transported thousands of miles. Apples are gassed with Methylcyclopropene which stops them ripening for 12 months and bananas for a month. Sulphur Dioxide does the same for grapes. What about freshness? Most supermarket items can stand on the shelf or in the refrigerator for weeks, or months, without spoiling. The preservatives enabling this are going into our bodies. That nice head of Broccoli in the store won't have any live enzymes and has been grown in nutrient-depleted soil and saturated with toxic pesticides. But who cares? It looks nice.

Government subsidies to mammoth corporations (who, due to revolving-door politics and campaign contributions, ARE the government) make grains cheaper than fresh fruit and vegetables. This, unfortunately, contributes hugely to sickness in society. Poor families cannot afford healthier produce and are left little choice but to eat low-cost, inferior-quality food. The Food Industry isn't at all embarrassed about poor quality. It tells us they are feeding us junk. We eat it and eat it, encouraged by a scary-looking clown, a bottle of bright red ketchup and artificially-coloured, sugar-water with bubbles.

Prior to the advent of large-scale farming, mankind ate fresh, living produce. Ripe fruit was eaten straight off the tree. Vegetables would be eaten shortly after being harvested, were grown locally and eaten in season. When I eat truly organic fruits and vegetables they are mouth-watering and delicious. Introduce them to someone addicted to junk food and they turn their nose up, or spit it out as 'tasteless'. Recently, I met a young lady with the usual problems... obesity, Type II diabetes, high blood pressure, constipation and high cholesterol. She had not eaten a vegetable in a year. "I don't do vegetables", she said. Her symptoms made that painfully obvious.

Sugar Belly

Many people have asked me how to get rid of belly fat? In early 2013, I conducted a trial (at least, that was my excuse). I have always been slim and trim and struggle to gain weight. One iced-Mocha coffee per day soon changed that. I don't normally drink coffee because it makes my head spin and keeps me awake. However, there is no denying these fancy coffees are delicious. After a few weeks I started to notice my waistline thickening. Then realized I was addicted. If I did not get my coffee, I missed it. After 9 months I switched over to iced tea. The waistline kept expanding. Within 18 months it had shot from 31" to 36", I had put on 9kg and my six-pack was now a burgeoning one-pack. This from one drink per day, with no granulated sugar.

The culprit was easy to identify, since nothing else in my diet had changed. While I would request "No sugar", vendors were still adding condensed and evaporated milk. I discounted the evaporated milk, since its sugar content is fairly low, which left the condensed milk. There are around 1000 calories in one cup of condensed milk. That is high but I was only getting around 100. This is insufficient to cause such dramatic weight gain. What kind of sugar could it be? Almost certainly it was Fructose Corn Syrup (FCS). A chemically-altered sweetener, now in widespread use. Why is FCS a problem? Well, glucose is a natural sugar which is easy to metabolize. Fructose is very different. The liver is unable to properly metabolize fructose and stores the excess in fat cells, for energy use later. The liver becomes fatty, first, then the stomach, then the rest of the body.

Dramatic action was called for. An 8-day, sugar-free, juice-fast kick-started the reduction of my waistline, purging whatever garbage had built up in my system and ending my cravings. [Read the chapter 'The 6 Tastes' to understand how to end sugar cravings without having to fast]. With the help of a diet of reducing foods, within 3 months, my weight had returned to normal.

What had I learned from my 'research'?

- Sugar is converted to fat.

- Excess fat did not cause my weight gain. SUGAR did.

- The sugar was HIGHLY addictive. This shocked me the most.

- In a body which struggles to gain weight, the weight gain was rapid. As if my body was unable to metabolize the sweetened milk at all. Plonking it straight into my stomach fat cells.

- I experienced severe leg cramps.

- Cravings for something sweet developed, shortly after eating a meal. (Hypoglycemia).

- The coffee/sugar combination made me jittery and often gave me heartburn. (Coffee is very acid-forming).

- If this could happen to me so easily, I understood why so many are obese.

I do not know, absolutely, which sugar was used. Manufacturers are sensitive about consumers knowing. Research indicates either High Fructose Corn Syrup (HFCS) or Aspartame (a chemical sweetener) are in condensed milk. My bet was on the former. HFCS is derived from corn. Due to subsidies it is cheaper than cane sugar. Food scientists have altered the structure of this compound and will not reveal how they make it. Dr Mark Hyman, an American physician, informs us...

'...The average American increased their consumption of HFCS (mostly from sugar sweetened drinks and processed food) from zero to over 60 pounds per person per year. During that time period, obesity rates have more than tripled and diabetes incidence has increased more than seven fold.'

In the United States, HFCS has become a sucrose replacement for honey bees. Beekeepers are putting HFCS inside the hives. The collapse of bee colonies has been linked to this dietary change. The sensible thing to do would be to withdraw HFCS from the market until we know it is safe. Producers think otherwise. Like the Tobacco Industry before it, they leaped into defence mode, with massive misinformation campaigns. Physicians were presented with 'science' showing HFCS was no different to other sugar. Professors of nutrition and experts from Harvard were recruited to spread the message to the public. Millions of dollars were invested. Next time you go to your Doctor and say, "Doctor. I think it's the fructose corn syrup making me fat. Should I eliminate it from my diet?" The Doctor will likely repeat the industry propaganda, "Sugar is sugar".

No it isn't. An alarming side effect was cramp. I would drink a sweetened tea, or coffee and, within an hour, be hit by an excruciating charley horse. The cramp was worst at night. I would fly out of bed, hopping and howling around the bedroom, trying to force my foot flat, on the floor, to relieve the cramp. Two glasses of hot water would eventually do the trick. At first I did not link the cramps to the coffee, because they also occurred after eating biscuits, then I found HFCS is a sweetener in biscuits. Since cutting out both biscuits and condensed milk, there have been no more cramps.

Another effect was cravings. 30 minutes after eating, I would feel a powerful craving for something sweet. This was new and troubling. Postprandial (after a meal) hypoglycaemia occurs when your blood sugar levels drop dramatically and the brain says, "Quick! I need glucose!" Hypoglycaemia is a prelude to full blown diabetes. I had taken it too far. So ended my addiction/experiment.

Aspartame

Another growing consumer worry is Aspartame. You may know it as Canderel, Nutrasweet, Equal or Spoonful. If you have not looked at the history of this sweetener, please do. The first thing to understand about Aspartame is it is not a natural sweetener like Sugar Cane, Maple Syrup, Honey or Stevia. It is a synthetic chemical, 200x sweeter than sugar, discovered by accident in 1965. The company that discovered it, G.D. Searle, were refused FDA approval until 1980, due to concerns about toxicity and brain tumours. However, when senior politician Donald Rumsfeld joined the board, Aspartame gained approval. Aspartame is now in 9000 products, worldwide, including chewing gum, yogurt, diet soft drinks, flavoured sports and energy drinks, fruit-juices, puddings, cereals and powdered beverage mixes. If you eat processed food it is virtually impossible to avoid it.

Why is Aspartame troubling? Every time you take in Aspartame you get a micro-dose of three poisons, two of which are known carcinogens - Formaldehyde and Formic Acid. The third, DKP, is a tumour agent. Aspartame-poisoning causes allergies and sensitivities and mimics diseases and disease syndromes. It is difficult to pin down the exact scale of the problem because most people with health issues will have no idea what is causing their symptoms. The largest numbers of complaints to the U.S. Department of Health are for headache, dizziness, depression, vomiting, abdominal pain/cramps, changes in vision, seizures and memory loss. **Dr Woodrow Monte, Professor of Food Science and Nutrition at Arizona State University** has studied Aspartame for 30 years and established direct links between Aspartame and several diseases, including cancer, heart disease, multiple sclerosis and Alzheimer's. In the UK, a University of Liverpool test-tube study found that, when mixed with a common food colour, aspartame becomes toxic to brain cells.

Trials, using Aspartame on rats, caused brain tumours yet it was still approved. Rates of brain tumours in children are on the increase. One small sign consumers are wising up to the danger, is Pepsi taking Aspartame out of diet soda. However, its replacement, Sucralose, is 600x sweeter than cane sugar. Out of the frying pan and into the fire?

A worrying new development comes from manufacturers seeking to sweeten milk and dairy products with these artificial sugars, without declaring it. If the GM soy milk you are drinking is sweetened with Aspartame and you are sickened by it, you will never know the cause because the ingredients will not be on the label.

Water, Water, Everywhere

Supermarkets do a great job providing a one-stop-shop for all our needs. So you would expect to see water, one of our basic needs, on the shelves. There are all kinds on offer. Mineral water, spring water, coloured water, flavoured water, water with bubbles, water from icebergs, kiddies' water. Once-free natural springs and water supplies have been bought up by giants like Pepsico, Coke and Nestle and sold back to the public.

There was controversy in the UK in 2013 when it was discovered 30% of store-bought bottled water came from the tap. Then even more when it was found bottled water cost more than milk. Business greed aside, what are the dangers in water? The list of possible contaminants is long. Fluoride, Chlorine, BPA (bisphenol A) from plastic bottles, endocrine disruptors, oestrogens, petrochemical pollution, micro-organisms, bacteria, farm run-off, chemical spills, pharmaceuticals and raw sewage. Bottled water is considered free of most of these. Bottled water can be stored for up to two years, during which time, levels of contaminants leaching from plastic bottles can build up. Sunlight and heat accelerate this process. Switching from bottled to tap water does not eliminate risk.

Tap water can contain high levels of:

Aluminium (implicated in Alzheimer's)

Lead (reduces intellectual development in children)

Iron (dangerous for babies and young children)

Diuron ESK (a pesticide which commonly exceeds safety limits in drinking water)

Trihalomethanes (linked to cancer and stillbirths)

E.Coli (a bacteria potentially deadly to babies and the elderly).

Fluoride

When it comes to breath-taking deceptions, there have been few as spectacular as Fluoride being 'good for your teeth'. Fluoride is a highly toxic industrial waste, poisoning workers, farm animals and land surrounding Aluminium plants. To understand the story of fluoride you have to go back to the 1930's and the aluminium and nuclear weapons industry. Fluoride (hydrofluorosilicic acid), is a by-product of aluminium production. It is not the natural element of fluoride. Industrial processes produced millions of gallons of this hazardous waste every year and massive amounts of fluoride were needed to develop the first nuclear bombs. Deceiving the public was deemed necessary, by powerful industrial and military chiefs, worried a tide of lawsuits would threaten the Manhattan Project (nuclear weapons program). Clean up costs for environmental contamination ran into thousands of dollars per ton. It became imperative to find a cheap way to dispose of this hazardous waste, convince the world fluoride was safe, and make a little money on it. In 1931, the Mellon Institute, at the heart of defending industry against asbestos claims, came up with the idea fluoride is great for our teeth and safe at low concentrations. Since 1945 it has been dumped into the water supply.

"If this stuff gets out into the air, it's a pollutant; if it gets into the river, it's a pollutant; if it gets into the lake, it's a pollutant; but if it goes straight into your drinking water system, it's not a pollutant. That's amazing." - **Former VP and Senior Chemist at the U.S. Environmental Protection Agency.**

Water fluoridation has been hailed as one of the "Top 10 public health achievements of the 20th century" by the U.S. Center for Disease Control (CDC). Yet World Health Organization data, from December 2014, reveals countries with the lowest rates of tooth decay do NOT add fluoride to their water supplies. 98% of Europe rejects water fluoridation.

The biggest concern is fluoride accumulates in human tissue. In Supermarket bottled water, labels do not state the concentration of fluoride. Consumers have no way of knowing if limits are exceeded. We absorb fluoride, orally, from bottled and tap water; toothpaste; baby food; soft drinks; cereals; beer; anti-depressants like Prozac and Paxil; dentistry; through our skin, via baths, showers and swimming. Fluoride is added to pesticides and herbicides, then sprayed on fresh fruits, vegetables and crops, which are also irrigated with fluoridated water. Maximum recommended levels of fluoride, for children, are exceeded by toothpaste, alone.

"Fluoride causes more human cancer, and causes it faster, than any other chemical... more people have died in the last 30 years from cancer connected with fluoridation than all the military deaths in the entire history of the United States [...] Fluoride amounts to public murder on a grand scale. It is some of the most conclusive scientific and biological evidence I have come across in my 50 years in the field of cancer research." - **Dr. Dean Burk, Congressional Record, July 1976**.

What led Dr Dean Burke to make such a dramatic statement? He took the 10 largest cities in the U.S. with fluoridated drinking water and the 10 largest cities without, then compared rates of cancer. He estimated 1 in 5 cancers was attributable to fluoridation. The WHO informs us fluorosis affects millions of people around the world. In Asia, skeletal fluorosis (too much fluoride) is endemic, known to cause irritable-bowel symptoms, hip fractures and joint pain. Confirmation comes from the **U.S. Department of Health and Human Services**, who state too much fluoride causes "chronic joint pain" and "arthritic symptoms." With 1 in 3 Americans suffering rheumatoid arthritis and osteoarthritis, the question arises, why have no studies been conducted comparing rates of arthritis between fluoridated and un-fluoridated populations? High fluoride concentrations in the pineal gland have been associated with early puberty in girls. Fluoride has been found to weaken the immune system and damage kidneys and liver. It destroys intestinal mucosa. Multiple studies show fluoride lowers IQ. The Communist Soviet Union added fluoride to prisoners' water, in concentration camps, to keep them docile. Anyone taking fluoride-based, anti-depressants soon learns about its doping effect on the brain and sexual function. When the pineal gland becomes calcified, by fluoride, it blocks our ability to reach higher states of consciousness.

Mustn't forget. Studies proving fluoride is good for teeth?

"No trials". "Unscientific". "Unproven".

"Neurodevelopmental disabilities, including autism, attention-deficit hyperactivity disorder, dyslexia and other cognitive impairments, affect millions of children worldwide [...] In 2006, we did a systematic review and identified five industrial chemicals as developmental neurotoxicants:

Lead, Methyl mercury (common in vaccines), Polychlorinated biphenyls, Arsenic and Toluene. [...] Since 2006, epidemiological studies have documented six additional developmental neurotoxicants- manganese, fluoride, chlorpyrifos, dichlorodiphenyltrichloroethane, tetrachloroethylene, and the polybrominated dihenyl ethers. We postulate that even more neurotoxicants remain undiscovered." - **UK Medical Journal, 'The Lancet'**

According to the **Centers for Disease Control**, 22 percent of America's children have dental fluorosis. Does this sound to you like a "Top 10 public health achievement"? The Union of EPA scientists reject fluoridisation of water.

'Recent, peer-reviewed toxicity data, when applied to EPA's standard method for controlling risks from toxic chemicals, require an immediate halt to the use of the nation's drinking water reservoirs as disposal sites for the toxic waste of the phosphate fertilizer industry'.

Still not convinced? In 1997 The FDA ordered a warning to be added to toothpaste labels. "If you accidentally swallow more than used for brushing, seek professional help or contact a poison control center immediately." They have since added another warning, advising children under 12 not to use it. 'Swallow' and 'poison' are two words that should not be in the same sentence. Why the so-called consumer protection agencies allow it, at all, when they acknowledge it is poisonous to under-12's is unfathomable. The warning is nonsense. If fluoride poisons the under-12's, it poisons ALL of us. Such a label only serves to demonstrate the power corporations have over the system. Never mind the harm, keep the toothpaste commercials going. We consider Fluoride such a serious risk to health we have designed a 'Fluoride Detox' program to remove it.

Where Does Supermarket Food Come From?

Today, giant food companies process, package and present most of the food we eat. Where do they source their produce? Traditionally, food came from small, decentralized, family farms. Today, it comes from concentrated, industrial-scale factory farms, requiring few workers. There is no longer a free market in agriculture. 'Agri-business' rules. Today there is only one buyer and one price. Enormous amounts of waste contaminate nearby water, with harmful levels of nutrients and toxins as well as bacteria, fungi, and viruses. The on-going takeover of millions of small farms and arguably the whole of agriculture, from seed to plate, by industrial-scale 'Agri-Business' and Food Processors, is a global health disaster, threatening an end to earth's rich food diversity. Does mankind really benefit from a handful of major corporations like Monsanto and Cargill monopolizing global agriculture and shaping it to their advantage? These two corporations have been labelled the 'thugs of big food'. According to critics, Monsanto has wiped small farmers in America off the map. They have shut down traditional seed cleaners, forced farmers to sell up or transfer their crops to Monsanto's GMO seeds and are buying up seed companies all over the world, leaving farmers with nowhere else to go and no choice but to use GMOs. Monsanto is the chemical company responsible for creating Agent Orange (used in the Vietnam War), PCBs, Roundup (glyphosate) and other toxins independent experts say threaten human health and the environment. To give you an idea of the character of this company, on February 22, 2002, Monsanto was found guilty of poisoning the town of Anniston, Alabama with their PCB factory, then covering it up for decades. They were convicted of negligence, wantonness, suppression of the truth, nuisance, trespass, and something I have never heard of before, 'outrage'.

Cargill touches almost every aspect of our food supply. In their inhumane **Confined Animal Feeding Operations (CAFO)**.

'Animals are crammed by the thousands, or tens of thousands, often unable to breathe fresh air, see the light of day, walk outside, peck at plants or insects, scratch the earth, or eat a blade of grass.'

Robert Martin, Director of the **Pew Commission on Industrial Farm Animal Production** had this to say:

"The present system of producing food animals in the United States is not sustainable and presents an unprecedented level of risk to public health and damage to the environment, as well as unnecessary harm to the animals we raise as food."

The risks he speaks of? More antibiotics are given to animals than humans. Overuse is resulting in bacteria becoming resistant to antibiotics, which is having a serious impact on the treatment of infectious diseases. Over-reliance on a single herbicide, glyphosate, is creating 'superweeds'. In 2012, 50% of U.S. farmers reported glyphosate-resistant weeds on their farms. More than 60 million acres. The problem is even greater today.

"The greatness of a nation and its moral progress can be judged by the way its animals are treated."

Mahatma Gandhi

Genetically-Modified Food

Imagine a world in which natural seeds are virtually extinct and the only commercial seeds available are genetically modified, patented and owned by one corporation. Wouldn't that corporation have tremendous pricing power and control over every nation on earth? Welcome to why Monsanto is one of the most feared and despised companies in existence.

What is it about GM food which causes so much concern? GM foods have been sold to the public based on five claimed benefits.

- They were needed to feed the world
- Have been thoroughly tested and are safe
- Increase yield
- Reduce the use of chemicals
- Can be contained and co-exist with non GM-crops.

All five benefits have been shown to be false. Ask the families of 125,000 Indian farmers who committed suicide after genetically-modified BT Cotton failed, what they think about increased yields? In 2009 a Union of Concerned Scientists report demonstrated that, in spite of years of trying, GM crops return fewer bushels than their non-GM counterparts.

Ask all those suffering from Chronic Fatigue, MS, Lupus, Allergies, Eczema, ADHD and other conditions, about the safety of GM foods? The number of people reporting to Doctors with these conditions has risen dramatically since the introduction of genetically-modified seeds in the early 1990's. **The American Academy of Environmental Medicine (AAEM)** has called on all physicians to prescribe diets without GM foods, to all patients. They stated,

"Several animal studies indicate serious health risks associated with GM food"

Including infertility, immune problems, accelerated aging, insulin regulation and changes in major organs and the gastrointestinal system.

"There is more than a casual association between GM foods and adverse health effects."

Ask the farmers, complaining to Monsanto about the failure of their herbicide to stop weeds, about reduced use of chemicals. A UK study showed canola cross-pollination occurring as far as 26 km away, demolishing the claim GM crops can be contained. Consumers around the world do not want GM foods until they have been demonstrably shown to be safe. Instead of providing proper safety checks, Monsanto has reportedly tried to force governments to accept GM products, by coercing, infiltrating and paying off government officials. As far as health is concerned, GM foods can be added to the long list of toxic foods to be eliminated from our diets.

Glyphosate & Health

Glyphosate ('Roundup') is the No.1 herbicide/pesticide used throughout the world. Despite this, few tests have been done to ensure its safety on humans and certainly no long-term studies. On June 12th 2013 a laboratory in Germany reported finding traces of glyphosate in the urine of 44% of adults in 18 European countries. Highest concentrations were in 90% of Maltese and 70% of Germans, Poles and Britons. More recently, glyphosate traces have been found in the breast milk of U.S. women, at levels suggesting accumulation in the tissues.

In another study, German researchers found '...chronically ill humans showed significantly higher glyphosate residues in urine than healthy population. The presence of glyphosate residues in both humans and animals could haul the entire population towards numerous health hazards.'

In March 2015, The **World Health Organization (WHO)** shocked the global biotech (GMO) industry by classifying glyphosate as a "probable human carcinogen". A 2014 study showed glyphosate is 125x more toxic than regulators stated.

"It is commonly believed Roundup is among the safest pesticides. . . . Despite its reputation, Roundup was by far the most toxic among the herbicides and insecticides tested. This inconsistency between scientific fact and industrial claim may be attributed to huge economic interests, which have been found to falsify health risk assessments and delay health policy decisions." – **R. Mesnage, Biomed Research International**

Occurrences of leaky gut syndrome, IBD, colitis, celiac disease and other chronic gut conditions have spiked since the onset of 'Roundup-Ready' GMO crops, which are reportedly disrupting the balance of our gut bacteria.

http://www.ncbi.nlm.nih.gov/pmc/articles/PMC3945755/

Gluten-Intolerant?

Gluten-intolerance has been blamed for numerous gut disorders. Yet, when sufferers eat grains imported from other countries, or eat the same grains abroad, they don't experience the same symptoms. What's going on?

A shocking farming practice, not widely known, which has become the norm over the last 15 years, occurs in the few days leading up to harvest. To reduce wear and tear on farming equipment, make harvesting easier and increase yield, wheat crops are drenched in Glyphosate-containing herbicides. How does this increase yield? As the plant dies it releases slightly more seed than it would do normally.

Considering traces of glyphosate are being found in chronic disease sufferers, it appears it is not intolerance to gluten we are seeing but intolerance to weed-killer. More studies have been called for to determine why weed-killer is being found in our bodies. For me, the question is not whether so much glyphosate is being found in human tissue but how do we get it out?

USDA Organic

I used to scan the Supermarket aisles for organic products. These were always more expensive than their non-organic brethren, yet that did not matter. My health and that of my family were worth it. No longer. The 'USDA Organic' label may have started out well but when Wal-Mart starts getting in on the 'Organic' act, it's time to question. Suspicions were confirmed when I discovered Wal-Mart, Safeway and Costco buy their 'organic' milk from factory-farms.

Large multinationals ('Big Food') bought up independent organic brands some time ago. That should not be a problem if they maintain organic standards. However, that is not what has happened. Major corporations have infiltrated the National Organic Standards Board (NOSB), the body recommending which substances are allowed and which are prohibited. 'Big Food' is now effectively setting organic standards and seeks to add more and more non-organic and synthetic products to the permitted National List. It seems the USDA 'Organic' certification has become just another way to seduce customers into spending more money for something which has little additional value. Inspection and regulation is so lax as to be worthless. Violations go unpunished. A good place for consumers to learn more is The Cornucopia Institute (find them online). Cornucopia keeps scorecards on all the organic providers as well as the performance of the NOSB. Having become wise to research trickery, I take industry propaganda which says, 'Organic is no more healthy than non-organic' with a pinch of Himalayan Sea Salt.

Food Corporations idea of 'organic' may have rendered the term meaningless but there are still many smaller organic operations who are trustworthy. I no longer put my health at risk buying 'USDA Organic'.

Food Corporations

Food companies, like any company, exist to make a profit. Seeking the lowest cost of production while charging the maximum price the market will bear. They also seek to establish monopolies. "Competition is a sin", tycoon JD Rockefeller informs us, establishing a corporate mind-set happy to destroy competitors and anyone who stands in the way of profit. Nations have been invaded and destroyed, solely for the benefit of 'Vulture Capitalism'. I will spare you the history lesson.

Corporations seek a competitive edge, constantly looking for new products or ways of improving the old. One challenge facing food companies is how to increase the shelf-life of food. Rotting food has to be discarded, costing the retailer. Therefore, wherever they can, manufacturers substitute natural, living, organic food (which degrades), with dead, synthetic chemicals coated in sugar, salt and fat. Made to look appealing. A good example is blueberries, found in cereals and cakes. They are made from artificial colours, hydrogenated oils and liquid sugars. The 'blue' in blueberry comes from a petro-chemical-derived colouring. Selections from 14,000 lab-made additives, with names none of us can pronounce, make food look fresher, more attractive and increase shelf-life.

NOTE: Two additives you may have encountered are called 'fruit' and 'vegetables'

Slick marketing tries to convince you industrialized food is no different to organic food. This myth is backed by hired food experts and one-sided 'Tobacco Science'. The media, long ago, abandoned investigative reporting and do not challenge industry propaganda unless activists and consumer groups force them to. One fast-food chain in the U.S. called 'Chipotle', seeing an opportunity, is enjoying strong sales. On 27th April 2015, it announced its policy, of abandoning genetically-modified ingredients in its food, is now complete. Chipotle has replaced GMO soybean oil with sunflower oil and is conducting trials to replace fructose corn syrup, in its root beer, with an organic sweetener. They still sell Coca-Cola but at least they are on the right track. The wrong track for some, it seems. Industrial sabotage is suspected as Chipotle products have recently been found contaminated with E-Coli affecting 12 States.

There is much more to reflect on, when discussing Supermarket 'food'. Such as frozen foods and pre-prepared meals, almonds which have been gassed and fruits that are waxed (how DO you remove that coating?!) I have barely touched on the ways the Food industry contaminates our food.

I realize much of what is written is indigestible but I hope you are becoming more conscious of the fact, 'There is No Food in a Supermarket'. If you believe there is, I would suggest your chances of recovering your health are pretty slim.

'Green' Advance

Some good news amongst the bad. If being 'refreshed' with radiation isn't perking up your rotting strawberries, it's recycling to the rescue. 70 million tons of food waste goes into UK landfill sites each year. The good news? Waste once thrown away by Supermarkets can now be recycled and turned into a source of profit. Want to compost your food waste? Say hello to home recycling composting units. These machines take your kitchen prep scraps, dining room table scraps and bones, uncoated paper/cardboard, and heat it to 180°F/82°C. This decomposes and deodorizes the mixture, while sterilizing seeds and killing bacteria. The entire process takes less than 24 hours and results in a 90% mass reduction. The dry output can be used as compost, bio-fuel, animal and pet food, while the extracted water can be used in the garden. If you are juicing fruits and vegetables day-in, day-out, as I do, you might enjoy such a machine. There is only one snag. Giving my pets cardboard to eat does not sound like a key selling point!

What is Real Food?

We have become divorced from our food. Where it comes from. The soil it is grown in. How it is harvested and prepared. Even how to cook it. Generations of youngsters are growing up having little experience of real food.

Here is what they are missing:

- Real vegetables are grown in balanced soil, rich in nutrients, containing all 52 trace minerals the body requires.

- Real fruit is tree-ripened, picked in season and eaten fresh.

- Real food is perfected by nature, safe to eat, tried and tested over thousands of years.

- Real Food can be used to PREVENT and CURE disease

- Fresh, live, organic food, eaten sensibly, will energize and invigorate you. Not cause obesity, diabetes, cancer and damaged arteries.

- Real food is organic and uncontaminated.

- Real food has many different varieties.

- Real food perishes within days.

- The soil real food is grown in is allowed to rest and recover. It becomes a haven for wildlife.

- Real food comes from animals which have been cared for, allowed to eat natural feed, and roam freely, in green pastures.

- Real food TASTES better!

Are you eating REAL food? If not and you wish to prevent or heal disease, it is time you did. But where to find it? If you live in the U.S. UK or Europe, chances are you will have organic food growers near you. They may be small organic farms, food cooperatives, local markets or individual smallholders. Prior to the 2008 recession, the organic industry in the UK was worth 1.7 billion pounds. Since then, sales have dropped as consumers have tightened their belts. If you have a patch of land or allotment, you may choose to grow your own food, from non-GMO seed, which is the cheapest way to do it. However, before you rush out and buy fresh celery and those juicy, tree-ripened apples, it is time to take a look at WHAT you should be eating.

Finding the Right Diet For You

An important consideration when it comes to food is our own unique, individual need. We are not all the same. Hence the saying,

"One man's meat is another man's poison"

Modern food production has created a global, integrated food chain where geography and climate no longer matter. Forget the seasons. You can eat imported Kiwi fruit and strawberries, year-round. Fast-food chains offer the same menu wherever you are in the world. Our bodies used to tell us what we are missing and what we should not be eating but these messages have been drowned out (or fooled) by nutrient-dense foods, sugar, tobacco, alcohol and coffee.

Knowing what to eat has become terribly confusing and complex. Battles constantly rage between celebrity dietary gurus. They are all sincere, educated and well-meaning and absolutely believe in their ideas, but goodness. Isn't it confusing? Should we be on low-fat or low-carb? Do we exclude meat, fish or anything with a face? Are we supposed to eat vegetarian with dairy, vegetarian without, or go 100% vegan? Is that cooked or raw? How is it my Chiropractor has a superb physique, looks incredibly healthy and claims he achieves this on a Fruitarian diet, yet, when I tried it I ended up weak as a kitten and my teeth nearly fell out?

What about a macrobiotic diet? The Japanese seem to do well on it. Should we 'Eat Right For Your Type' or be on the Mediterranean Diet? Pasta washed down with a couple of glasses of red wine? Surely I should be eating the foods growing in my geographical area, most suited to the climate? How can an Eskimo survive on raw, leafy greens? Can he even find them? What happens if I move from a cold to a hot country? Have you tried eating salad during a North European or North American winter? Do I eat what I was raised on, or is it best to go 'native'?

The number of diets is bewildering. There are hundreds of them. The latest is the 'Paleo' diet, a diet our ancestors are said to have consumed. Do we listen to Dr. Loren Cordain, who penned 'The Paleo Diet' and says we should get protein from meat? Or to T. Colin Campbell, who wrote 'The China Study' and says we get enough protein from plant food, and animal products promote Cancer. How do you decide, when both present persuasive arguments? It is certainly complicated.

What I do see is no serious natural healing protocol advises you to cure your disease with a rump steak, unless it's a black eye. They all say 'BUY A JUICER!!' and 'Get those live, green, healing juices into your bloodstream!' My pet dog

'Juicefast' agrees. When sick, he goes out and eats leaves and grass. He is after the chlorophyll. We may have forgotten how to heal ourselves but animals know instinctively. Whether it is cows licking clay, monkeys eating leaves to expel parasites, or cats eating houseplants. Animals in captivity sicken and die because they are prevented from doing this.

Yet, hold on a minute. My grandmother used to make hearty bone soups to build us up and fortify us against colds and the flu. Chicken and bone soups were a household staple, with pulses, garlic, ginger, onion, potato and vegetables. We are supposed to strengthen our immune systems, aren't we? Today's factory-farmed animals are not as healthy as when grandma was alive and I would not consider using them for healing. Nonetheless it is a fact humans have been eating meat for 2 million plus years, while degenerative diseases didn't start appearing until about 150 years ago, around the same time refined grains and refined vegetable oils were introduced. Every year the Standard American Diet includes more of these foods, triggering increased obesity and disease. Is meat really to blame?

The use of animals for fortifying the immune system, or building the emaciated, is not confined to colder, northern countries. Have you ever seen a black chicken? In Hong Kong, an elderly Chinese healer, alarmed at my emaciated state, cooked me a stew with black chicken, Chinese herbs and spices. She was adamant that, if I did not follow her advice, I would be dead in a year. When I tried to inform her I do not eat meat because I was juice-fasting I was met with a withering look which said 'Have you completely lost your mind?'

The British Royal Navy Field Gun crew are some of the toughest, fittest men in the world. They need a diet which gives them power, endurance and speed. I never saw one eating salad. It was always meat, raw eggs and milk. Yet Olympic champions like Carl Lewis claim their best performances came on a vegan diet. It is too early to observe which diet benefits their long-term health but Carl Lewis reports what I found during my 4 years on a vegan diet. Feeling lighter (not just in weight terms), and cleaner.

Major studies have been done comparing the health of meat-eaters and vegetarians over time. The news has not been good for vegetarians. In Feb 2014 a study of Austrian men came to this startling conclusion:

'Austrian adults who consume a vegetarian diet are less healthy (in terms of cancer, allergies, and mental health disorders), have a lower quality of life, and also require more medical treatment.'

'Studies have shown a vegetarian diet to be associated with a lower incidence of hypertension, cholesterol problems, some chronic degenerative diseases, coronary artery disease, type II diabetes, gallstones, stroke, and certain cancers. A vegetarian diet is characterized by a low consumption of saturated fat and cholesterol, due to a higher intake of fruits, vegetables and whole-grain products. Overall, vegetarians have a lower body mass index , a higher socioeconomic status, and better health behavior, i.e. they are more physically active, drink less alcohol, and smoke less. On the other hand, the mental health effects of a vegetarian diet or a Mediterranean diet rich in fruits, vegetables, whole-grain products and fish are divergent. For example, Michalak et al. report a vegetarian diet is associated with an elevated prevalence of mental disorders. A poor meat intake has been shown to be associated with lower mortality rates and higher life expectancy and a diet which allows small amounts of red meat, fish and dairy products seems to be associated with a reduced risk of coronary heart disease and type 2 diabetes. Additionally, evidence concerning lower rates of cancer, colon diseases including colon cancer, abdominal complaints, and all-cause mortality is, however, inconsistent.'

Such conclusions are weakened when you consider some will have adopted the 'healthier' diet because they were already sick. Nevertheless, it was a major shock to the vegetarian and vegan world.

I spent several months in Kerala, a State in the South West of India, which is a vegetarian and vegan food lover's paradise. You would think the Keralan population would be pretty healthy. Yet I was struck by the number of overweight people I saw even in the rural villages. Vegetarians and vegans are typically slim. In June 2014, a systematic review of 142 articles found hypertension rates across India, including Kerala, running at around 25%. This increase coincided with the replacement of natural oils and sugars, with refined.

The conclusion I draw from all this is we are omnivores. Our bodies will utilize whatever fuel we provide it with. At least in the short term. I have met those who thrive on a vegan diet, those who thrive on a vegetarian diet and those who thrive on a diet high in animal products. I have also seen the converse. Over the longer term, food not suited to our constitution is toxic.

The question of what is the right diet for us is crucial. The question of what to eat when sick is VITAL. Food nourishes and sustains us. Hospitals and Doctors make a grave error not understanding nutrition and not knowing the patient.

Different foods grow in different geographical regions and various methods of growing, harvesting and preparing food have evolved. In non-industrialized countries, food is largely uncontaminated. In industrialized nations, it may take a little more effort but pure food can be found. How do you decide what to eat? Some eat to live. Others live to eat. How food looks, tastes, feels ('mouth-feel') and smells is important. Is it light or heavy, warm or cold, oily or dry? Is it emotionally comforting or energising? 'Variety is the spice of life'. Is your plate interesting and varied or are you eating the same meal every day? Is your meal balanced?

I once took a 6-month trip in a van through 12 countries in Europe. I threw a futon in the back, a small gas cooker, and off I went. I won't bore you with my adventures but I did notice, as I traversed each country, the different body shapes, kinds of foods and local eating habits. I spent a week in Riga, the capital of Latvia, and was struck by the fact that, in 7 days, I did not see one obese person. The food they eat was direct from farm to table. Latvia does not allow GM foods into the country. Nobody took any special steps to stay slim. It was just a normal consequence of their diet. Russia was the same, so was Poland, Lithuania and Latvia. The soil in these regions is rich. There is no monoculture. Crops are varied. Overall health has deteriorated in these countries since my trip 15 years ago. More so, after the 2008 financial crisis. Poverty has deepened and social economic factors are largely to blame. Clearly there is a lesson there. Eat a variety of fresh, uncontaminated, nutrient rich foods. By eat I don't mean over-eat!

We are mainly made up of water. Like a swimming pool our body PH needs to be balanced. Not too acid and not too alkaline. Around 7.35 (slightly alkaline) is normal. Foods can be either acid-forming or alkaline-forming. When I grew up, a balanced meal was meat and two vegetables. The meat is acid-forming and the vegetables alkaline-forming. Now the vegetables have been replaced by french fries, doused in ketchup and washed down with a chilled soda. All acid-forming. That acidity has to be neutralized to maintain the PH. The body does it by taking calcium from our bones. Naturopathy considers Acidosis (too much acid) a significant health problem, causing numerous disorders. I think this is generally true but, like everything else, it gets complicated. In '**The Rainbow Diet**', Chris Woollams informs us some people become more acid after eating meat, while others more alkaline. What!

Life used to be simple. Not anymore. Reductionist science means we know more and more about food and yet it seems, 'The more we learn the less we know'. We know about vitamins, minerals, phytochemicals and antioxidants. We know about acid/alkaline balance. We know about blood types, metabolic types and constitutional types. Food scientists and nutritionists discover more each time I research the subject. Scientists make discoveries, only to change their minds a few years later as each new discovery emerges. Like a troupe of French Can-Can dancers, they flit across the stage, flick up their skirts and shout 'Voila!' Our titillated hearts skip a beat but after you have seen them enough times, scientific 'discoveries' no longer impress.

In 1973, the **American Heart Association** recommended limiting egg intake to a maximum of three eggs per week. An idea picked up and echoed by health experts. The UK took it further, advising a maximum of two, even though mankind has been eating eggs for thousands of years. Why? Because 'bad', 'bad' eggs contain artery-clogging cholesterol. Health officials ended up with egg on their chin, when cholesterol in eggs was found to have almost no effect on blood levels of cholesterol. The research group gave government officials a lesson in nutrition, saying,

"Egg is a cheap food that is rich in very high-quality proteins, minerals, folates and B vitamins. Thus it can provide a large quantity of nutrients necessary for optimum development in adolescents."

The policy was shelved. Small comfort to egg producers who went out of business.

A HUGE dietary change which has almost certainly led to many deaths and diseases is the myth saturated fats = coronary heart disease. For decades Doctors and the media told us saturated fat was bad for us. Refined oils, fats and margarines killed off natural oils and spawned the multi-billion dollar, low-fat food industry. Cancer and heart disease have exploded since the switch from butter, lard and natural oils to refined oils, homogenized glop and trans-fats. The anti-saturated-fat dogma gave 'Big Food' the perfect excuse to wean us off foods which had sustained us for centuries (portraying them as natural born killers) and move us on to more lucrative, nutrient-deficient, processed products, stuffed with chemicals and cheap fillers. What did food manufacturers replace the lost fat with? Sugar.

In March 2014 a UK Cambridge University study was published in the Annals of Internal Medicine, called '**Do Saturated Fats Really Cause Heart Disease?**' Data was collected from 72 previously published studies of more than 600,000 people, from 18 countries. The conclusion? Saturated fats do NOT cause coronary disease. The fact mankind has been consuming saturated fats, such as in coconut oil, for thousands of years, without any adverse health effects, seems not to have entered the minds of food scientists, or the public. Replacing saturated fats with industrial oils did not reduce the risk of heart disease. It increased it. What did the research say reduced cardiovascular disease? Margaric acid, found in dairy fat!

There are other examples of State Health 'Can-Can' girls falling head-first into the orchestra pit but you get the idea. Listening to official government advice can make you sick. These defenders of the nation's health, in deed, if not in word, appear to be working on behalf of corporate food giants and not the public they claim to represent.

Like global warming, the science surrounding food is not settled and is used to confuse instead of enlighten. Arguments are still raging today, over diet, almost 100 years after the first diet craze, triggered by Doctor Lulu Hunt Peters '**Diet & Health: With Key to the Calories**' book, published in 1918. For me, it is better to ignore the 'froth and bubble' of these experts, until they sort it all out, and stick with the simple lessons the ancients taught us. As my good friend Dr Paul

Johnson reminds me… 'there is nothing new under the sun'. A key to understanding diet remains the classic theory of the "humors" – warm, cold, moist and dry – believed to exist in every substance and organism. Illness was believed to derive from physiological imbalance and a simple, natural diet was the best method for re-establishing it. Spend a month eating only McDonald's and you will quickly understand physiological imbalance.

Ayurveda & Diet

Ayurveda means 'Science of Life'. It is a 5,000 year old holistic, personalized, traditional healing system, with over 400,000 registered practitioners, fully supported by the WHO and Indian government. Other traditional healing systems, like Traditional Chinese Medicine (TCM), Thai Traditional Medicine (TTM) and Tibetan Medicine, are all derived from Ayurveda. Ayurveda offers detailed individualized guidance on food, nutrition and diet, based on your Constitutional Type.

[For explanation on Ayurvedic Constitutional Types, see Appendix]

Dr Richard Schulze, from the **Thomsonian School of Healing**, is adamant the best diet for health is a whole food, vegan diet. From someone who has cured thousands of patients of the most serious diseases, he would surely know. Yet, I did not thrive on this diet. When I look at him, he is a large-framed, heavy-set man with adequate fat stores. A classic 'Earth' type. This type does well on a light vegan diet, since it acts as a counter to their natural tendency toward heaviness. If Richard was eating heavy, high-calorie foods, he would gain weight quickly. Clearly with so many people experiencing obesity this diet is well-suited to them, since they are 'reducing' foods. I, however, am a slim 'Air' type. The opposite to Richard. My frame is small, light and dry. 'Air' types need grounding, with warm, heavy, oily foods. Light, vegan foods are detrimental to their health. I probably made some mistakes but basically, what is good for Richard Schulze is bad for me and vice-versa.

If you have intestinal disease, food sensitivities or an inflammatory bowel disorder, it is hard to build mass because you may not be absorbing nutrients from your food, no matter which diet you are on. According to the Kelley Metabolic Diet (a sophisticated system of identifying the right diet), my type can pretty much eat anything. Except, when it comes to healing from chronic disease. Then a lighter, cleansing diet may be appropriate, for a period. The deciding factor is the strength of the person. If you have little excess fat and are emaciated, you need to be properly nourished with 'building' foods which support healing, before considering lighter foods. It is important not to leap into a raw food program or juice fast, without first assessing the ability of the person to undertake it.

The Six Tastes

When it comes to diet, most people's level of understanding comes down to how food tastes. It is probably the most important consideration in deciding what to eat. But what do we really mean by 'taste?'

The ancients understood there is more to food than calories, and developed, over time, a sophisticated understanding of the properties and actions of food and how it can be used for prevention and healing. This knowledge has been lost, or forgotten, in the West. A very important property of food is taste and I don't mean just the taste sensation in the mouth.

There are 6 tastes in nature:

Sweet

Sour

Salty

Bitter

Astringent

Pungent

Each of these 'tastes' has important effects on body and mind. The Standard American Diet (SAD) is heavily dominated by three. Sweet, Sour and Salty. Food Corporations know we do not like bitter tastes, so saturate processed food with excess sugar, salt and fat. The other three tastes are essentially missing. Our taste buds have been trained to salivate over these three tastes and reject fresh fruits and vegetables which become 'tasteless'. In fact, if you have tried supermarket fruit, it IS tasteless.

'Sweet', in particular, is highly addictive. Ever tried to eat just one biscuit from a packet? Biscuits are banned from our household since none of us can eat just one. The whole packet is gone in minutes. Manufacturers add appetite stimulants which make you want to eat more. They also use sophisticated tests to identify the 'Bliss Point'. This is the exact measure of sugar, fat and salt to excite your taste buds and brain. Neither too much, nor too little. Junk food is purposefully designed to stimulate this Bliss Point. Millions are addicted.

How can we break this food addiction? The most important of the 6 tastes is 'Bitter'... Bitter melon, dandelion, bok choy, kale, cabbage, broccoli, water cress, bitter herbs and many more. Sour and pungent (spicy) foods have a place but are less important. What is so important about 'Bitter'?

- Bitter stimulates a sluggish liver and improves detoxification. (Dandelion is a classic liver tonic).

- Eliminates food cravings. Bitter turns off Sweet!

- Thins and purifies the blood. It is antibacterial, anti-viral and anti-fungal

- Resets the taste buds

- Reduces fat

- Is a laxative

- Is anti-inflammatory.

You can see how important this taste is. For weight loss, detoxing, health and healing; and how, by not including it in our diet, it can lead to a whole heap of dietary trouble. I call the bitters my 'Clean-Up Crew'. I have observed, in the north of Thailand and villages of Southern India, villagers sharing a meal, sitting cross-legged on the floor. They each have a plate, or banana leaf, with meat, fish or rice. Other plates/banana leaves are filled with a variety of dark green, bitter leaves. Villagers are not pre-occupied with hygiene (most have no concept) and rely on the protective power of bitters (and hot chillies!) to deal with any pathogens. Although physically smaller than their growth-hormone-eating western counterparts, these villagers are strong, slim and can work all day on rice farms, under a tropical sun. I do see some smoking and drinking of alcohol and sugary sodas (Thais put sugar in everything), yet northern village Thais do not put on weight, as their urban counterparts do. The 'bitters' are protecting them. It is only when they abandon these protective foods cancer, heart disease, diabetes and obesity rates accelerate.

How Can We Use the Six Tastes for Healing?

If you are serious about restoring your health, it is important to do two things. Eliminate foods designed to get you addicted; introduce 'bitter' into your diet, and create your own 'clean-up' crew! Every food has an associated 'taste'. If you know what these are, you can use this knowledge for healing.

There is an art to it but I will keep it very simple:

REDUCE

Sweet, Sour, Salty

INCREASE

Bitter, Astringent, Pungent

To a certain extent, natural healing programs do this already. **The Gerson Therapy**; Richard Schulze's 'Incurables' program; Retreats, like ours. Authentic detox programs include dark, leafy, bitter greens in their juices. Most people have heard of Wheatgrass Juice. In India, Ayurvedic bitter combinations are used for healing and to cure diseases such as Cancer. In Kerala I sampled one particularly bitter mixture and, boy oh boy. No matter how much I knew it was healing me, I vomited, it was so potent. Bitter drinks can taste 'vile' to western palates conditioned to like sweet. The good news is, once your body is cleaned up and taste buds reset, you can tolerate them more easily. In fact, you may find yourself vomiting when you go back to the sugar! For softies, like me, bitters can be mixed with sweeter juices, like carrot, apple or beetroot, to make them more palatable. As Mary Poppins warbles:

"A spoonful of Stevia helps the medicine go down... the medicine go dow-own..."

Tourist-focused healing spas and resorts, understandably, don't like to see customers emptying the contents of their stomachs into the ornamental gardens. Forget those bitter herbs. Their 'healthy' juices tend to be Coconut, Pineapple and Mango shakes with a sprig of mint and a colourful mini umbrella. It probably won't heal you but you will enjoy a pleasant holiday.

"You cannot build a house to last 100 years using poor quality materials. Nor the human body."

Paul Keenan

The Hidden Qualities of Food

If you are unwell and desperately want to feel better, it is understandable you turn to experts. Unfortunately, they present so much complex, confusing and contradictory advice I would understand if you threw your hands in the air and followed the nearest group of lemmings over a cliff. It is exasperating, to say the least. My answer to this vexing situation is to turn to the ancients, who are not encumbered by the minimalistic complexities of 'science'. What we learn from the ancients is simple and clear.

While studying Ayurveda, I learned why 4 years on a vegan diet had left me cold, emaciated and without energy. And why the following 3 years, on a vegetarian diet, did the same. I learned the food I was eating was hindering my recovery, not helping it. Depressing my immune system, not strengthening it. Depleting my resources, not building them.

What else did the ancients teach me? That, besides The Six Tastes, food has other actions on the body which can be recruited for healing. That foods can be:

Heating or Cooling

Drying or Moist/Lubricating

Building or Reducing

There is more. Some foods have an 'inward' energy and some an 'outward' energy. Some 'upward'. Some 'downward'. I had never heard of this but considering it, realized the ancients were right. If I eat ginger, blood flows to my hands and feet (ginger has an outward + heating energy). If I eat a banana, my hands and feet become cold (bananas have an inward + cooling energy). I am perhaps more tuned into it but give it a try.

How is this useful? If you are a smoker and have Peripheral Arterial Disease and need to get blood to your extremities, why not recruit ginger for the task? Or chilli, which is a vasodilator (widens the arteries). We have all experienced the heating power of chillies. Mix horseradish, ginger and mustard powder, stick it in your socks (Not against the skin!). 'Phew!' If that does not get the blood flowing to your extremities, nothing will. There are products like Capsicum (Chilli) plasters which encourage this, in most pharmacies. Spas and massage shops have 'heating' balms which draw the blood to the skin or induce sweating.

If you are a fiery, ginger-haired, freckled Scotsman with eczema, diarrhoea and heartburn, forget the chillies. You are way too 'hot' and need cooling down. Cold showers, salads, dairy and refrigerated foods and drinks can help.

If you are overweight, lethargic and tend to retain fluid; introducing spicy and drying foods such as salads, hot spices and diuretic herbs, is the way to go. They will increase your metabolism, reduce your weight, dry out excess mucus and increase fluid excretion.

Circulatory disorders kill more people than any other cause, worldwide. So, it is not such a bad idea to include heating or warming foods in your diet. Ask Fauja Singh who, aged 100, became the oldest marathon runner in the world, what he thinks of ginger? He credits ginger curry, ginger tea, low stress and a vegetarian diet as the secret to his long life. Vegetarian and Vegan diets are certainly healthy for the right person in the right situation. However, some people do seem to have problems with vegan diets. I met quite a few on my spiritual/health travels who looked emaciated and anaemic. Larger-framed types do well on them but slender 'Air' types, as mentioned previously, need nourishing, building and grounding. A vegan diet is wrong for them. Idealistic vegans will argue strenuously over such a view, believing everyone can be strong and vital on such a diet. However, when you probe, their strong line is usually due to concerns over animal welfare and defence of their own choice. For those who are overweight or obese, a 'reducing' vegan or vegetarian diet is generally recommended.

The question of 'WHAT TO EAT?' for each individual is not yet clear. There is an everyday diet and a diet for healing. Sometimes they can be the same and sometimes not. For chronic disease, a period on a strict healing diet is often a necessity.

"Let food be your medicine and medicine be your food".

When considering a healthy eating plan, there are some minimum requirements. Food should be:

Fresh

Uncontaminated

Locally grown

In season

Unprocessed.

Nutritionally dense/nourishing.

Incorporate all 6 tastes.

Varied

Colourful (eat the rainbow!)

We need a diet to maintain health, or reverse disorders, which takes into account our individual reactions to food. These can determined by tests such as Applied Kinesiology, VEGA testing, the RAST test, the Coca Pulse test or observing our own reactions to food (sneezing, gas, bloating, runny nose, canker sores, excess mucus, constipation, heartburn, diarrhoea and vomiting).

There are numerous suggestions from various camps as to which diet is best suited to our particular type. I will mention four:

- USDA Food Pyramid

- 4 Diets for 4 different Blood Types, as suggested by Peter J. D'Adamo

- Metabolic Typing introduced by William Donald Kelley. This identifies if you are a vegetarian, carnivore or should be eating a balanced diet.

- Diet based on your Ayurvedic Constitutional Type

The USDA Food Pyramid, heavily influenced by industry lobby groups, has been discredited. Many Americans following it have gained weight and become sick. Eating diets based on your Blood Type is also suspect and was the subject of an article published in Jan 15th 2014 in PLOS, an online medical literature site. The article said:

'...the present study is the first to test the validity of the 'Blood-Type' diet and we showed adherence to certain diets is associated with some favourable cardio-metabolic disease risk profiles. [...] However, the findings showed the observed associations were independent of ABO blood group and, therefore, the findings do not support the 'Blood-Type' diet hypothesis.'

In other words, if you eat a healthier diet you will benefit but this has little to do with your Blood Type.

With a claimed success rate of 93% in curing newly-diagnosed cancer and a 50% claimed cure rate for those who have undergone conventional treatment, the **Kelley Metabolic Typing Diet** ranks highly. Based on answers given to approximately 130 questions, you can identify the right diet for you.

I like Dr Kelley's methodology and accuracy but for simplicity, the Ayurvedic Constitutional Type system of 'Air', 'Fire', 'Earth' and 'Water' has as much going for it as any other system, with a far longer track-record. No system I have tried, explains my characteristics as well. This does not mean it will be the same for you or other methods are better or worse. You need to try them and see which is the best fit, for you. Where I would adjust a diet is by taking into account individual reactions to specific foods. The diet you eat for your Constitutional Type should serve you well, except where you experience adverse reactions. Then, you need to eliminate these foods, either for good or for a period, then re-introduce them, to see if you can tolerate them once more.

If you need an example of the difference a change in diet can make, look no further than Novak Djokovic who, on the 12th July 2015, won the Wimbledon Tennis Championship, beating Roger Federer. Novak altered his diet to eliminate gluten products and credits this and other dietary changes for his incredible endurance, vitality and speed.

Many people have an intimate relationship with their food. Food lovers have a difficult time making changes. They cannot stop thinking about food, talking about food, dreaming about food and eating food. They LOVE food! For those who 'live to eat' it is clearly more difficult to change their diet than for those who simply 'eat to live'. For everyone, it is crucial to enjoy the food we eat. However, what do you do when the food you love is slowly poisoning you? It is not complicated. Change your diet or stay sick. You decide.

The Five Layers of Healing

8 Steps To This... 7 Steps To That... 10 Things You Absolutely MUST Do Before...

'How-To' lists are never-ending. I can barely remember 3 steps when someone is giving directions. Yet, it is worth paying attention to certain health 'How-To's'. When trying to understand what may be out of balance in an individual, practitioners have to be like detectives. A super method exists to help identify where an imbalance may lie which helps focus healing efforts on the RIGHT rather than WRONG area.

In the 1980s Dietrich Klinghardt is credited with developing a systematic model called '**The 5 Levels of Healing**'. Based on ancient understandings of Body, Mind, Emotions/Energy, Spirit and Intuition. The idea is disease, or imbalance, can occur any or all of these layers. (You may have heard of 'psychosomatic'. The mind affecting the body.)

Chronic and degenerative disorders can involve any or all of these 5 levels. My view of Klinghardt's model is slightly different, simplified and based on the Ayurvedic view of the individual. To distinguish between the two methods, I call them Layers instead of Levels.

- The **Body Layer** is our physical body, including our senses. Allopathic medicine operates on this level.

- The **Mental Layer** is our thoughts, attitudes and beliefs. Psychiatry operates on this level.

- The **Emotional Layer** is our feelings, which in reality is also the Mental Layer, since all feelings are preceded by a thought. Whether we love, hate, laugh or cry, experience regret, guilt or shame.

- The **Energy Layer** is primarily our autonomic nervous system, which can be upset by trauma, chronic stress and electro-magnetic fields. It includes our 'Aura'. A field of energy which radiates from a person.

- The **Spiritual Layer** is the connection between you and 'God', whatever your conception of 'god' is. It is the intrinsic part of you which never changes. The observer. The charioteer. The 'Self' or Soul. The part of you which transcends body and mind.

The Spirit Layer is also the area where past lives, generational effects, spirit beings and 'Karma' prevail. Whether you believe in these or not does not matter as far as your healing is concerned. It is not necessary to accept everything. Only keep an open mind and stick with your program.

The western world accepted Body, Mind and Spirit, long before atheistic, mechanistic forces decided to attack religion and 'murder' the Soul. The success of the merchant class in moving the masses away from worship of God, to worship of the material, has left tens of millions with no concept of the Soul, Self or Spirit, beyond worshipping their favourite football team and celebrity 'false gods'. We have been conditioned to look outward and not inward. To gratify the 5 senses. To 'just do it'. To not look to the Church 'family' for guidance and wisdom but the corporate or collectivist State. People no longer know themselves. They have lost touch with the 'Self'.

When it comes to approaching the topic of spirituality, many people are closed. Believing religion is responsible for most of the world's ills. Without considering it is the individuals at the top who have hijacked and distorted religions, for their own nefarious purposes. The usual culprits, power and wealth. Also, most people do not distinguish between religion and spirituality. The best alternative practitioners are sensitive to individual's feelings on spirituality and use language and techniques which allow them to approach the subject without 'spooking the horses'. Better yet, simply leave the topic alone and allow inner transformation and spiritual awakening to take place, naturally. As it often does during the process of healing.

The following examples, of how The **Five Layers of Healing** can be useful, start with Ben.

The Geordie 'Guru'

Ben, from the North-East of England, was (he claimed) something of a celebrity 'Guru' in California. Being English gave him an advantage. Americans love the British accent. He wore a black Fedora hat, an amulet round his neck and talked the Yoga talk. Ben had a relaxed, easy-going 'Geordie' manner. When I chatted with him, in my garden, I could see Ben wasn't what he seemed. While knowledgeable in some practical aspects of Yoga, it became clear to me he knew nothing of Ayurveda and little about health. Somewhat strange, since Yoga was a fundamental part of Ayurveda.

Ben looked like a drinker. His weathered face carried the signs. His admission his girlfriend was an alcoholic made me wonder if Ben, himself, was drinking. When, during our conversation, he lit up a cigarette, claims to being a Guru evaporated in a puff of smoke. It was disappointing. Like encountering devout worshippers for two hours on a Sunday, who then go home and beat the kids.

It would be unkind and unfair to call Ben a hypocrite. Any knowledge which helps people should be commended. Yoga is a useful discipline, especially in healing. Iyengar Yoga, a good example. However, as with so many I meet, Ben still had work to do. Yoga had not really cured him.

A Gluttonous Priest

Choking with emotion I sat, spellbound by the most wonderful sermon, delivered in a picturesque English village Church, by a huge, bearded bear of a man, with shining visionary eyes. The congregation were all weeping, such was the power of this man's message.

"Yes!" We all wanted to be like Jesus.

"Yes!" We were absolved of our sins.

"Yes!" We embraced each other, joyfully, as brothers and sisters.

For a moment, the congregation were transported out of their mundane, stressful existence, to a better place, seated at God's right hand. This inspirational prophet had affected me like no other. His deep, warm, compassionate voice made me feel secure. I was captivated and moved. So when he asked my wife and I to join him, at his home, for Sunday dinner, we both eagerly accepted. At last, I thought. Here is someone I can believe in.

Such thoughts evaporated, once we sat down to eat. The meal was laid out before us, a typical English Sunday Roast. I had never met a glutton before. Gluttony is one the Christian Church's **7 Deadly Sins**. Bits of half-eaten food and gravy fell and coursed through his beard, as the priest tucked in. He cleared his plate quickly, polished off the extras, then moved on to his wife's unfinished plate. I looked on in barely-concealed astonishment. I did not know then but understand now, this 'man of the cloth' was under tremendous strain. The effort and desire to be like Jesus. To be whom the congregation wanted him to be. To live in accordance with his own inspirational words. It was all too much. The priest needed an outlet for his stress. He found it in food.

The Path of Knowledge

Standing on the platform of a bustling, Indian train station, surrounded by thousands of people, I looked toward the approaching train. Suddenly, my eyes were drawn to a bald, white head, bobbing up and down in the crowd facing, not toward the train, but in my direction. Something told me this individual was going to track me down and sit next to me. Sure enough, five minutes after boarding, a young man dressed in spiritual garb came into my carriage. I do not recall his name or even if he gave it.

"Mind if I join you?" he asked.

"Please do." I replied.

With shaven head and eager expression, the young man sat opposite and started to speak. Non-stop, he talked about religious history, philosophy and spiritual practice. His knowledge was incredible, his grasp of the subject, undeniable. We swept through the countryside, missing the sights and sounds of village life, as he spoke. Every now and again, I nodded and smiled but did not interrupt. After three hours, the young man's batteries ran out. He stopped and looked at me, a tad self-consciously.

"Goodness", he said. "I have been talking all this time and you haven't said a word. You seem very calm. Tell me. What do you think the most important Spiritual practice is?"

I paused for a moment, looked him in the eye and said, "Silence".

It was one of those moments which live long in the memory and I chided myself for being so rude. Yet the young man's reaction said it all.

"Oh my God", he exclaimed, somewhat embarrassed. "You are right. You are right."

Of course I was. This man needed to be quiet. To empty a mind, filled to overflowing with knowledge, leaving no room for self-reflection and the inner work which was really needed.

Conclusion

What do these three examples tell us about the 5 Layers of Healing? Well, first of all we can clearly identify some of the layers.

Ben, the 'Guru' had chosen the PHYSICAL Layer as his path to wholeness.

The hungry Priest had chosen the SPIRITUAL Layer as his path to salvation.

For the walking library that was the religious devotee, it was knowledge. The MENTAL Layer.

Ben needed Spiritual power to overcome his addiction to alcohol.

The Priest needed to Mentally surrender and accept it is impossible for anyone to 'be like Jesus'. (I have observed young Catholic missionaries and trainee priests suffer breakdowns, attempting to be like Jesus).

The young Hare Krishna had deeper problems. The Path of Knowledge is a legitimate route to 'self-realization'. Academics, intellectuals and thinkers are naturally drawn to this path. However, he needed Emotional healing. His eyes were telling me, "I have all this knowledge. I know all the spiritual practices. Yet I am still suffering. What am I missing?"

I hope you are beginning to see how helpful this way of looking at people can be. How understanding the 5 Layers helps identify where the root cause of a problem may lie.

These are examples of individual Layers. What about multiple Layers?

Angela

At the age of 12, Angela was a gifted gymnast, good enough to represent her country at the Olympics. Physically and mentally operating at optimum performance. When her parents divorced, Angela fell into a deep depression and started comfort eating. Her weight gained, she was constantly fatigued and her gymnastics career was effectively ended. By the time she was 24, Angela had seen many Doctors and Psychiatrists, in an attempt to lift her depression. Nothing helped. After meeting and talking with her I had a feeling as to what was wrong and asked if she had tried the 'Spit Test'?

The 'Spit Test' is a 'quack'-hunter's dream. The idea is that, when you wake in the morning and before you put anything in your mouth, work up some sputum, then spit it into an 8oz glass of water. According to the theory, if you have an overgrowth of Candida (also known as thrush/yeast/fungus), the sputum will form 'Jellyfish legs' which descend toward the bottom of the glass. These legs are colonies of yeast, clumping together, forming strands. The longer the legs, the more systemic the Candida. Angela was absolutely classic for systemic Candida overgrowth.

[Please do not rely solely on this test. There are around 80 possible symptoms of yeast infection, which help confirm a diagnosis. Many online sites provide free Candida questionnaires].

Learning fungi thrive on sugar, Angela opted for a 10-day, sugar-free juice fast. 10 days is the length of time needed to kill fungus in the body, with fasting. Angela could have tried commercial anti-fungals but they carry risk and are not always effective. Angela had colloidal silver and an herbal (anti-fungal) tincture, as part of her regime. Angela felt more tired than usual, throughout her fast, with neither energy, nor desire, to leave her bed. Our retreats offer Yoga, meditation, swimming, sauna, massage, health education and more. Angela wanted none of it. She asked me if she should get up? I encouraged her to listen to her body. For the next ten days Angela rarely left her room, except for an EFT/NLP session to dissolve negative feelings relating to her parent's divorce. It was clear something was happening, as white strands of dead fungi were being eliminated from her bowel. This was the cause of Angela's additional weariness. It is called 'die-off'. When fungi in the body start to die, they release toxins into the bloodstream. A variety of symptoms, usually not serious, can manifest. Tiredness is one.

By the 11th morning, when Angela had completed the program, she was still very lethargic and down. Dragging herself out of bed, she needed to get back to normal life and join friends for a holiday in Bali. Many people who undertake juice fasts feel fantastic around the 5th and 6th day. With raw food programs it is the same but can take a little longer. This did not happen with Angela. The experience for her had been draining. You could understand if she left with negative feelings about juice-fasting. Yet, three days later, Angela contacted me.

"I feel amazing", she said.

Angela's depression had lifted and she felt "totally energized!" Feeling so well, in fact, she persuaded her friends to join her on a 10-day detox in Bali. She quickly followed that with a 12-day detox with her grandmother, back in Canada. Last I heard, Angela had a new career selling health supplements (quality supplements, I hope, Angela!)

When someone is in a deep depression they are unable to come out of, more than one Layer is involved. Christian thinking believes chronic depression is a psychological problem with a Spiritual root. Angela was certainly affected at the Physical and Emotional levels. Her parents' divorce had depressed her immune system. Side effects of anti-depressants and/or antibiotics may have added to her physical problems, causing dysbiosis (microbial imbalance in the gut). Providing an opportunity for Candida to gain a foothold.

I have the utmost admiration for Angela. When the temptation to do so must have been tremendous, she never quit.

"Each morning lean thine arms awhile upon the window-sill of heaven and gaze upon the Lord. Then with that vision in thy heart, turn strong to meet the day"

Thomas Blake

Breaking The Chains

'Breaking The Chains' is a powerful, simple, visualization exercise I use to address the Emotional and Spiritual layers. The belief is, our attitudes and behaviour, today, can be negatively influenced by past events, sometimes going back generations. For instance: If, a century ago, a family member was murdered (or committed murder) the effects of that event can be passed down through subsequent generations. Perhaps through anger, guilt, family shame. Likewise the death of an infant; war; suicide, etc... 'Breaking The Chains' is used to end the influence of these past events. It can also be used to address current issues. To,

"Break the chains that bind us".

Let's say you have fallen out with a parent and not spoken for years. It may be their fault. It may be yours. You want to resolve the situation but pride, fear or stubbornness prevent you. You may be too angry, or ashamed, to face them. Or you have moved to another locality or country. You may feel they would never accept an apology or offer one. This applies equally to others, not just a parent. Sisters, brothers, grandparents, aunts, uncles and cousins. You can expand the list to include a difficult boss at work, a deceased child, soul-mate you are still grieving over, the man who violently raped you, friend who tricked you of your life savings, the ex-wife or husband you are still sore at, or the childhood sweetheart who callously dumped you for another woman. Whoever you have hurt, or who has hurt you.

It is important to understand we must forgive, to liberate ourselves. Yet many times we cannot. When we think about people who have hurt us, it is painful. We cover our hearts in psychological concrete, lock the past away in our mental cellar and ban any mention of their name. Understand. These issues do not go away. They still affect us. Do you really wish to take bitterness, or sadness, to the grave? In what way is this helpful to you? Do you not realize holding on to pain, fear, anger, shame, remorse and regret, may be contributing to your poor health and preventing recovery?

The Church understands the power of the Confessional. Other religions have similar devices. There is no approval or disapproval. No judgment. Only the desire to liberate you from your chains. The cause of your pain may no longer be alive, may not live near you, or you may lack the courage, or opportunity, to face them directly. 'Breaking The Chains' gives you that opportunity. To face them all in role-play and get whatever is upsetting you off your chest. Visualize that person standing in front of you and imagine them apologizing, or giving you their blessing. Whatever the situation merits. Your intuition will guide you. The imagination is powerful and can, even if you think it cannot, picture them in front of you.

Ask a trusted friend, family member, or even a stranger, to play the role of the person you wish to speak to. Or if you feel uncomfortable, sharing your deepest feelings with others, take some blank sheets of A4 paper, write down the first letter of the person you have issues with… 'M' for mother, 'F' for father, etc… and so on, then spread them around the floor. Go to each one in turn and talk to them. It can be helpful to have someone with experience guide you but if no-one is available, do it yourself. You will soon get the hang of it. Very often people do not know there is a problem until they start talking. Many times, incidents we have suppressed, or forgotten, come up.

Have some compassion, too, for the object of your pain. THEY may also be suffering regret, guilt, shame, anger or fear. THEY may wish to have their pain dissolved but do not know how to do it. Once you have liberated yourself, liberate them too. Go and see them and tell them how 'Breaking The Chains' liberated you. They may reject your approach but that's ok. You have done what you can.

Sceptics love to criticize techniques like this but who cares what they think? Your only concern should be, does it work for you? If success is due to the 'Placebo Effect', celebrate! If it is because it is the first time you have really faced the issue, terrific! Often times, when helping others, I do not know exactly what worked or why it worked. Who cares? Be happy it HAS worked.

Breaking The Chains is a 'must-have' in any Healing Toolbox.

Craig

Craig was a humanitarian worker, carrying out dangerous work in war zones. He had almost lost his life on three occasions. When I met Craig he had been in and out of therapy for five years and was on anti-depressants. As the stress of his job increased, issues he had locked away in his mental cellar, started coming to the surface to be resolved. This is a very common phenomenon with stress. One incident, in particular, was troubling him.

Twenty-three years previously, Craig's one-year-old son had died of bacterial Meningitis. Craig watched him die and could do nothing to save him. Being young, he was able to have other children and move on quickly with his life, thinking time had healed the wound. It hadn't. Craig began to experience profound sadness and turned to alcohol to numb the pain. He lost interest in caring for himself, his diet was poor, he stopped exercising and his weight ballooned. This is when I met him.

One of the keys to Craig's recovery was 'Breaking The Chains'. Initially, Craig did not have faith in this exercise, in part because he was an introvert and did not look forward to the role play. However, he committed to trying everything because he genuinely wanted to feel better. During the exercise, Craig shared his innermost feelings to four key family members, living and deceased, with whom he had unresolved issues. Much to his surprise, the process became cathartic for Craig. That night he had vivid dreams that brought to the surface many forgotten memories. The exercise helped him move beyond unresolved issues and put things in perspective.

For Craig, there was a conflict between understanding he was not directly responsible for his son's death, and the emotional insistence that, as a father, he was responsible for his son's health and wellbeing. Many victims of trauma irrationally take on guilt in such circumstances. If the trauma is not fully processed, the guilt will fester and eventually surface in unhealthy ways: drinking, drugs, violence, insomnia, nightmares, irritability, and so on.

Another key to Craig's recovery was EFT. When Craig began the Tapping exercise he had to stop because he became too emotional. After the second tapping session, the guilt had dissolved. The memory of his son's death would always remain but the emotional pain associated with it was gone. Craig was able to put things in perspective. For the first time, he concluded he had four other lovely children who were alive and deserved his full attention and focus. Over the next few days he reached out to all of them and committed to cherishing and loving them and being part of their lives.

Cleaning up Craig's body, the Physical Layer, from the effects of alcohol and the sickness-inducing Standard American Diet, was also part of his recovery. A cleansing juice-fast has a rapid, transformational effect on every level. A Homestay Retreat interrupted Craig's drinking and isolated him from temptation and distraction. Flooding his body with nutrients, along with moderate exercise, had him feeling better, within days.

Craig's was a work in progress. He relapsed a few times but the retreat experience led to the confidence and knowledge he could be the Master and not the Slave of his cravings. In fact, so pleased was Craig with the outcome, he flew his daughter in, from the U.S., also to attend a Homestay. Today, some five years after the end of the program, Craig believes he has healed. He views the program as the turning point in his recovery and identifies the forty-five minute session of Tapping, as the single exercise which eradicated the irrational guilt over his son.

"Before the session, it was there. After the session, it was gone," he says.

Craig is no longer depressed and on medication. He hasn't had a drink in nearly four years, exercises five or six times per week, eats well and has lost 40 pounds. He enjoys his family and has become a healthy part of his children's lives.

Which of Craig's 5 Layers were affected? Physically, his nerves were shredded, his diet poor, he was overweight and had stopped exercising. Psychologically, he knew he was harming himself but did not know how to lift his sadness. Energetically, his nervous system was over-stimulated and exhausted. Emotionally, the memory of past events was causing him pain.

Craig believes that, although he was drinking heavily, he was not an alcoholic. Confirmation of this comes from the ease with which he was able to resolve his issues. Hard core alcoholics usually need Spiritual Power to overcome their addiction, which is why Alcoholics Anonymous makes the Spiritual Layer the foundation of their program.

"There is No Cure"

It may surprise you when a Doctor says, "There is no cure", he is being honest. He is just missing part of the sentence: "To my knowledge…"

Before I go any further, a quick reminder. Doctors work wonders with acute and emergency conditions. We absolutely need the skill and dedication of these medical professionals. However, Doctors know, for chronic, degenerative disorders, the current system does not work. Doctors are ignorant of alternatives. They simply do not know. This lack of knowledge seems odd in light of the fact healing systems like Traditional Chinese Medicine and Ayurveda have been treating and curing people for thousands of years. Why don't doctors know about their best practices and successes? Do they really believe the positive aspects of natural healing have already been incorporated into conventional medicine? Do Doctors really believe natural methods have never cured, or are unable to cure, anybody? Do they really believe when they have written off a patient who later returns, healed, that patient is lying? That they never had the disease in the first place?

If I were to ask a Natural Healer the same question, I would receive a very different response:

"Yes, you can be cured. If you are prepared to make the effort".

Why the difference?

The **Conventional Doctor** provides relief, is lost without a diagnosis, ignores individual variability and fails to address underlying cause. He has made up his mind what the problem is within three minutes of seeing a patient. He attacks the disease with methods which are toxic and invasive.

The **Natural Healer** treats the whole person. Seeks to identify and resolve underlying cause and his methods do not depend on a diagnosis. He or she gives time to understand the patient. He strengthens the patient, using safe, non-invasive methods.

Note: When I use 'Natural Healer' you can substitute any practitioner successfully using non-drug, non-toxic, non-invasive healing methods.

"The natural healing force within each of us is the greatest force in getting well."

Hippocrates

How Difficult is it to Cure Ourselves?

Over the last 150 years, there has been a profound change in our attitude to medicine. I would estimate, today, 98% of people have been conditioned to see a conventional Doctor if they are unwell. The other 2% will tackle their ailments themselves, or not at all. We go to our Doctor for the slightest ache and pain and gobble up antibiotics like sweets. Are people right to seek the aid of physicians?

Do you know the story of King Charles II? Fourteen of the highest physicians in the land are earnestly 'reviving' the King from a stroke,

"The king was bled to the extent of a pint from a vein in his right arm. Next, his shoulder was cut into and the incised area was sucked of an additional 8oz of blood. An emetic and a purgative were administered followed by a second purgative followed by an enema containing antimony, sacred bitters, rock salt, mallow leaves, violets, beetroot, camomile flowers, fennel seeds, linseed, cinnamon, cardamom seed, saffron, cochineal and aloes. The king's scalp was shaved and a blister raised. A sneezing powder of hellebore was administered. A plaster of burgundy pitch and pigeon dung was applied to the feet. Medicaments included melon seeds, manna, slippery-elm, black cherry water, lime flowers, lily of the valley, peony, lavender, and dissolved pearls. As he grew worse, forty drops of extract of human skull were administered, followed by a rallying dose of Raleigh's antidote. Finally Bezoar Stone was given. Curiously, his Majesty's strength seemed to wane after all these interventions and as the end of his life seemed imminent, his doctors tried a last ditch attempt by forcing more Raleigh's mixture, pearl julep and ammonia down the dying King's throat. Further treatment was rendered more difficult by the king's death."

You may be forgiven for thinking it was hundreds of years ago and irrelevant to practices existing today and yet, wasn't the use of ammonia then, the same as the use of chemotherapy, now? Chronic degenerative disorders could not be cured by King Charles physicians, nor by today's medicine (they tell us this themselves). This means 100% of us are wasting our time going to the Doctor for a cure. Relief? Perhaps. Cure? No. So why do we go and see Doctors? We can cure ourselves, if we only know how. How difficult can it be?

Of all the great healers I have researched, there is not one whose reputation, methods and successes have not been disparaged, or dismissed, with an airy wave. The charge of choice is that claims of healing are not supported by scientific evidence. They are all 'charlatans' and 'scoundrels'. I hope I have shown this charge to be bogus and much of conventional medicine and psychiatry have no scientific basis. So what did the great healers do? Many great healers become so after being healed of their own 'incurable' disorders.

Dr Sebi

Dr. Sebi was born Alfredo Bowman on November 26, 1933 in the village of Ilanga in Spanish Honduras. He never attended school and came to the United States as a self-educated man, having been diagnosed with asthma, diabetes, impotence and obesity. He weighed 291lbs. After unsuccessful treatments with conventional doctors, Sebi was led to an herbalist in Mexico. Healed of all his ailments, Alfredo was inspired to become an herbalist. Creating natural compounds, designed for cleansing and revitalization of all cells which make up the human body. His approach to healing with herbs was shaped by 30 years of practical experience.

Much has been said and written about Dr Sebi but what struck me about him was the inescapable fact he was cured and he was adamant juice and water fasting were KEY to his cure. In 1988 a case against him, for 'practicing medicine without a licence', was thrown out by the Supreme Court, when 70 witnesses swore Sebi's methods cured them of a wide range of disorders, including AIDS. What were those methods? Sebi fasted for 57 days, believing mucus is the major cause of disease. Eliminate mucus-forming foods from your diet and you will heal. This idea is not new.

Arnold Ehret

100 years ago, Arnold Ehret wrote about his Mucusless Diet Healing System. Few people today have heard of Arnold or his system. Arnold taught college until he was drafted for military service. After nine months he was released because of 'neurasthenic heart trouble'. He resumed his teaching career at 31, despite chronic ill health, suffering from a kidney disorder and Tuberculosis (TB). Under the care of 24 different physicians at one time or another, Ehret eventually turned to natural methods, vegetarianism and mental healing but without completely satisfactory results. A stay in Nice, living on a milk-and-fruit diet, was only partially beneficial. The following winter, Ehret traveled to Algiers. Living almost exclusively on the plentiful native fruits. His condition rapidly improved and he was emboldened to try short fasts, trying to aid the cleansing properties of the fruit and the climate. Not only did Arnold regain good health but also unbelievable energy, strength and joy of living. He and a companion undertook an 800-mile bicycle trip from Algiers to Tunis, returning completely exhilarated.

Dr Richard Schulze

'Dr. Schulze is one of the foremost authorities in the world on natural healing and herbal medicine. He holds a Doctorate in Herbology from the **School of Natural Healing** and a Doctorate in Natural Medicine. Dr. Schulze also holds a degree in Herbal Pharmacy and degrees in Iridology. He is certified in eight different styles of "body therapy" and has three black belts in the martial arts. Dr.

Schulze has written numerous research papers on the topics of Botanical Pharmacognosy, Pharmacology and the making of herbal preparations.'

When Dr Schulze was 11, his father died in his arms, of a massive Heart Attack. At 14, his Mother died from the same. They were both 55. At 16, he was diagnosed with a genetic, 'incurable', heart deformity. Rather than accept a similar fate, Richard worked hard on healing himself with lifestyle changes. Step-by-step, over a 3 year period, Richard repaired his heart.

Inspired to learn everything he could, Richard studied under the great healers. Dr. John Ray Christopher, America's greatest herbalist of the last century; Bernard Jensen; Paavo Airola and Dr. Kurt Donsbach, the renowned nutritionist. Richard took on thousands of patients, with the most serious diseases. His reputation grew until officialdom violently shut him down. In his book '**Common Sense Health and Healing**' Richard says,

'My clinics were open, spanning three decades, over 20 years, with over 20,000 patient visits in this country and abroad.

In the last decade of my clinical practice I specialized in degenerative and life-threatening diseases. Especially the ones medicine says are incurable, like cancer, AIDS, heart disease, arthritis, diabetes, liver and kidney failure, Alzheimer's disease and other neurological diseases.

The news of my success with these patients and their life threatening diseases spread. My clinical success became an embarrassment to the medical community, and my patients thriving instead of dying became embarrassing living testimonials to the failure of modern medicine. I was arrested and my clinic was boarded up.'

Richard Schulze's Wiki page was apparently deleted by a conventional Doctor. An indication of how much he threatened (or offended) the establishment.

There are countless examples like these, of famous healers, as well as testimonials from ordinary people, attending fasting retreats and spiritual centres, suffering chronic illness who, having been let down by conventional medicine, healed themselves using natural methods. Their stories offer hope.

Dr Sebi fasted for 57 days. Richard Schulze's Incurable program is 30 days, with a minimum of 12 days fasting. Arnold Ehret ate only fruit. All three were on diets which rested the digestive system, releasing vitality for healing.

Richard Schulze's observation was 80% of people were healed just by properly cleansing the bowel. This involves fasting and bowel cleansing. If fasting is not for you, you can achieve the same outcome, albeit more slowly, on a raw vegan or fruitarian diet.

You Cannot Heal a Dirty Body

By now, you understand, in natural healing, there are two main causes of disease. Toxicity and deficiency. Therefore, to bring about healing, it is necessary to remove toxins (clean the body), and provide adequate nutrition.

Why does the body need to be clean? According to cancer specialists, Max and Charlotte Gerson, as well as the great healers, "You cannot heal a dirty body". There are many ways to clean the body. The most common methods are physical and breathing exercises, steam sauna and massage, dry skin brushing, cleansing juices, raw or juiced vegetables, hydration, contrast bathing, liver and kidney flushes and bowel cleansing. Let's look at them, briefly.

Physical exercise gets the blood and lymph moving and opens up the pores, excreting toxins through the skin. Waste gases are expelled via the lungs.

Breathing exercises flood the body with oxygen and 'prana'.

Herbal steam saunas open up pores and raise the body temperature (high temperatures kill off pathogens and liquefies impacted waste).

Massage helps release and mobilize toxins, moving them towards the elimination channels.

Dry skin brushing removes dead skin layers and invigorates, while moving the lymphatic fluids.

Fruit Juices hydrate, cleanse and nourish nerve tissue and cells.

Contrast bathing is one of the best ways to get the blood moving. Repeatedly switching between hot and cold water, will at first bring fresh blood to the surface of your skin, then drive it deeper. The improved circulation helps deliver herbs or juices to areas of congestion.

Some cleansing programs are gentle and some more aggressive. For instance, you can encourage elimination of waste with gentle laxative teas or uniodized sea salt. Castor oil, Epsom salts and enemas are also effective. During the 'Master Cleanse' you drink two litres of salt water, within 40 minutes, which will flush the bowels rapidly. One Yoga cleansing method I sometimes undertake involves drinking 32 glasses of warm, salt water, two glasses at a time, followed by five different yoga stretches. This forces salt water into every nook and cranny of the colon. Diverticulitis (bowel pockets) is a common problem today. A 6-monthly routine takes around three hours and is a serious workout and cleanse.

The word 'Detox' is plastered on just about everything these days. Commercial 'detox' kits and teas can be found in most stores. Care needs to be exercised. i.e. You don't want to be taking in traces of chemicals used to bleach herbal tea bags.

Ayurveda has a thorough cleansing protocol, called 'Panchakarma', which uses heat, therapeutic massage, warm oil treatments and enemas, to liquefy and mobilize toxins and excrete them. Some sceptics do not believe toxins exist. They are convinced the liver detoxifies everything. Such people are either being too literal or their knowledge is out of date. The U.S. CDC (Centre for Disease Control) has identified hundreds of chemicals found in human and breast tissue and published the fact. Some worried mothers have turned away from breast-feeding, to infant formula, out of concern. Except infant formula is also contaminated and lacks the protection breast milk provides. When you mix infant formula with tap or bottled water you are exposing your infant to fluoride. Breast-feeding is still the best way to nourish and protect the new-born.

Pregnant women's unborn children are at serious risk from at least 12 developmental neurotoxins we know of and more we do not. According to researchers, a 'silent pandemic' of chemical contamination is occurring, on a global scale. What are these toxins? Chemicals like DDT, BPA (from plastics); heavy metals like mercury, lead and aluminium; poisons like fluoride and arsenic; parasites; fungi; bacteria; by-products of poor digestion; acid wastes; 'electrosmog' (radiation from mobile phones, computers, electrical devices and nuclear testing); even recreational and pharmaceutical drug residues. In a healthy person, these should be cleaned up efficiently and excreted. In someone whose health is compromised, they can accumulate and be backed up or stored in body fat. Some studies show, with the sheer number of pollutants in the environment, even the fit have around 500 different chemicals detectable in the body.

Sceptical minds do not understand physical toxins are not the only toxins. We also have toxic thoughts, toxic emotions and toxic relationships. It is common to use the word 'detox' to encompass them all. Remember the 5 Layers? Holistic practitioners see all as being in need of 'detoxing'. Not just the physical layer.

Proper **hydration** is crucial. Think of a dirty sponge. Leave a dirty sponge in a bucket of cold water, overnight. The next morning the sponge is clean and the dirt sitting on the bottom of the bucket. Same principle with us. Ordinarily we should be taking in enough clean water, via drinking and from fruits and vegetables, to allow proper hydration and elimination. However, most of us are not taking in sufficient fluids and are dehydrated. Contaminants and metabolic waste products are thus not mobilized and expelled. These find their way to the small capillaries, such as in our joints, where they lodge, causing inflammation and degeneration. During a detox, we flood the tissues with fluids and using manipulation (massage) and agitation (exercise), mobilize and move waste towards the channels of elimination. Cleansing programs like the **Gerson Therapy** or the **Master Cleanse** (Lemonade Diet) require you to drink fluid every hour, throughout the day.

A tip about massage. Many massage therapists are really only 'oil-smearers'. This is inadequate. You need muscles, nerves, lymph nodes and tissues to be kneaded and pressed. When I go for a Thai Traditional massage, the masseuse asks if I would like soft, medium or strong pressure? "None", I say. "Give me a savage beating". I am half-serious. I want FIRM pressure. As much as I can tolerate. I am not there to relax but to break up crystal formation, clear congestion and improve circulation. Keep this in mind. If you cannot find affordable, effective massage, have friends or family do it. We all know instinctively what to do. Who doesn't love a head massage? TRY. Your Doctor certainly isn't going to put his hands on you.

"The soil is our external metabolism. It must be free of herbicides and pesticides or the body cannot heal."

Dr. Max Gerson

Will We See Cures Soon?

From corporate-influenced medicine? The industry wants us to believe cures are always 'just around the corner' but do not hold your breath. While there are encouraging signs some mainstream Doctors are open to alternative viewpoints, for a conservative health industry to suddenly become trailblazers and bring cures to us, is as unlikely as arsonists coming up with proposals to extinguish a blaze they started. It is not going to happen.

Pressure for change has to come from the bottom-up. This pressure is set against entrenched and powerful vested interests, whose profit models, control and very existence, depend on the maintenance and expansion of disease.

"Last year, 75 percent of the $2.6 trillion the U.S. spent on health care was for treating chronic diseases that, to a large degree, can be prevented or reversed through lifestyle change" - Dr Dean Ornish

$2.6 trillion. That's astonishing. With a number like that, it explains why so few, beyond the patients, are interested in cures.

Sickness is a business and Cancer the biggest business of all. 70 years and vast amounts of money and research since the 'War on Cancer' was launched and they still do not know what causes cancer (so they claim). They force the same deadly treatments on patients, as decades ago and refuse to entertain or properly investigate safer alternatives. It is a strange system which crosses its fingers in the hope the cancer dies before the patient and in which shrinking (not eliminating) a tumour is lauded as a 'success', even if the patient dies. Earlier diagnosis is good. Better treatment. That's good. More sophisticated surgery. Good. Except, the survival time of a cancer patient is no greater today than it was fifty years ago.

In the absence of cures from mainstream medicine, the patient has to look elsewhere. Due to the monopoly power of the Medical-Industrial-Complex, 'elsewhere' is limited to CAM methods, which they know are of limited therapeutic value. We are forced to travel abroad or fix ourselves.

That's ok. We can do it. We are in the Bypass Age.

Medical Complexity

The practice of modern medicine is horrendously complex, producing a multitude of separate specializations. Depending on your health challenge, you may see an endocrinologist, cardiologist, neurologist, oncologist, rheumatologist, etc. You are passed from one specialist to another, none of whom may talk to each other and each of whom will have their favourite drugs. In theory, you can create a multi-system approach (dare I say 'wholistic') from these different disciplines. However, in practice, this would not work, since they still avoid underlying cause. The cocktail of drugs, you receive, will never have been tested in combination and will increase the likelihood of serious side effects. I do wonder why we call them 'side effects'? An effect is an effect. How do we know if the 'side effect' isn't the main effect?

On my first visit to Asia I was shocked by the number of drugs patients are given and the grossly inflated prices charged in hospitals. GPs and pharmacies dispense antibiotics with wild abandon. The poorly educated population can't seem to get enough of them. The lack of knowledge of 'side effects' is troubling.

The problem with the micro-management of disease is you get lost within the specialization. Does recovering one's health really require highly complex and fragmented specialties? During my time as patient and observer in one of India's 'Nature Cure' Centres, I saw no technology at all. No fragmented disciplines. Patients were being cured modern hospitals had rejected as 'incurable.'

The scientific method is increasingly being applied to natural and alternative medicine. New terms arise such as 'bio-resonance', 'bio-cybernetic medicine' and 'quantum healing'. **German Biological Medicine** has the most advanced concept of natural healing, today. Simon Yu, MD described it thus:

'German Biological Medicine integrates modern medical science with traditional European natural medicine, with a strong emphasis on homeopathy, biological terrain analysis, understanding the concept of pleomorphism, and integrating the philosophies of Traditional Chinese medicine and Indian Ayurveda medicine. It covers many different forms of natural healing including emphasis on mind/body and spirituality'.

I don't know about you but I was lost at 'biological terrain analysis' and 'pleomorphism'. While the German concept may be the pinnacle of what is available, and I applaud its integrative, holistic approach, most of us do not have access to it, cannot afford it and do not understand it. What benefit can there be in confusing the patient? This only makes them dependent. Healing needs to be simple. If you do not understand what a practitioner is telling you, you are less likely to apply yourself to recovery and are going to experience stress. A practitioner has an obligation to ensure a patient knows what is being done to them. I want to know what these people are giving me, and why? Those who come to me for advice, leave, knowing exactly what they need to do and why they need to do it. My '**Keenan Biological Medicine**' System (just kidding) is a bag of healing tools, extracting only those methods from Ayurveda, Nature Cure, Yoga, Qigong, EFT and Breaking The Chains which are simple to understand, easy to apply, and effective.

Simple or Complicated?

When faced with a wide choice of remedies available, which do you choose? I find it helpful to imagine a sliding scale, measuring from 1 to 10. 1 being the simplest remedy and 10, the most complex. Water fasting would certainly qualify as a 1, with German Biological Medicine being a 10. Academics and intellectuals will naturally be drawn to the more complex methods. Lesser mortals, to the simple. Water Fasts, historically used for healing across many nations and centuries, are as simple as you can get. Perhaps why over-educated Doctors are sniffy about them and we don't pay them much attention. It seems too simple. We like to be impressed by technical terms and science.

My own approach, in every possible circumstance, is to seek simplicity and avoid the horrifying complexity of mechanistic, medical reductionism. Macro instead of Micro. Gross instead of Subtle. Simple instead of complex. Natural and instinctive instead of Scientific and mechanistic.

In 2002 I was suffering arthritis in my knuckles, knees and toes. Like my mother, the prognosis was poor. After 44 days of massage with Sesame oil, a vegetarian diet and two bowel cleanses, my circulation was restored and joints pain-free. (I have seen similar results within 10 days on our detox retreats). My Ayurvedic Doctor did not speak a word of English, so I was spared any medical jargon. On the complexity scale, I would put his methods down as a 4. Gandhi's 'Nature Cure', which I also tried, might be a 2.

Coming back to the question 'Are you one of the 98% that can cure yourself?' According to the great healers, the answer is a resounding "Yes!" If you have the knowledge, are sufficiently motivated and stop violating the Laws of Nature. If your situation is not urgent, you have time to investigate solutions. You may start with simple, before moving up the scale. Cancer patients, told they may have only weeks to live, may reflect on the accuracy of what they are being told. They almost always have more time than they think. Time which can be spent exploring safe, non-toxic alternatives. Even where a Cancer is not being cured, practitioners can often stop the cancer from growing, by preventing the formation of new blood vessels. Which will buy you more time.

Modern Medicine vs Alternative

A Naturopath, in Europe, once took a drop of my live blood and put it under a Darkfield microscope. Looking at the screen, he made some interesting observations. Firstly, red blood cells are supposed to be circular, separate and bouncing off each other. Many of mine were clumping together. This is called platelet aggregation. Secondly, most of my red blood cells were teardrop-shaped, indicating prolonged stress (nature has a sense of humour). Thirdly, a majority of cells were pulsing in their centre. I was told this was a parasite. Finally, white crystals could be seen, which the Naturopath pronounced was my Arthritis. This all sounded plausible. Later I mentioned these observations to a conventional Doctor.

"Rubbish", was the verdict.

"All of it?" I asked, taken aback.

"All of it", he said, emphatically.

If I was suffering a chronic or degenerative disorder, today, and seeking advice on alternatives (complementary or natural healing) methods, the last person I would talk to is a conventional medical Doctor. What is the point? It is like asking someone who supports Manchester United football team what they think of Chelsea.

Industrialized, standardized, 'scientific' medicine, for the masses, cannot and does not provide holistic, tailored, natural treatments to individuals. Modern medicine sees little value or reward in 'old' medicine and has replaced the Art of Healing with 'Standard Practice'. Deviate from this and a Doctor can find himself in serious trouble. Patients have to accept some responsibility for this. As long as we remain satisfied with relief and are unwilling to change our disease-inducing ways, the health system is not going to change. Why should it? Corporations' prime concern is to make money and they do it very well. The top 5 pharmaceutical companies make more in one year than the whole continent of Africa. Profits from disease are stupendous. Profits from no disease are?

Arguments people have online, over Modern vs Alternative medicine, are brutal, never-ending, exhausting and irreconcilable. This battle has been going on for over 100 years. Non-conventional defenders have a difficult time of it because they are increasingly up against paid medical 'trolls'. What is a Medical troll? These are people (sometimes whole departments) tasked with patrolling the internet or sitting on health forums, disparaging and discrediting proponents and discouraging you from trying Alternatives. They 'run interference' on alternative topics and disrupt discourse.

There is much that is unsatisfactory about Alternative Medicine. 90% of Over-The-Counter (OTC) remedies and supplements are essentially useless. Many Alternative therapies will not cure (at least individually) and much of the Alternative Health Industry, like any capitalist enterprise, is built upon marketing. However, don't throw the baby out with the bathwater. There are authentic healers out there who know what they are doing. You just haven't encountered them yet.

My attitude toward health is not an either/or choice, embracing one method at the expense of others. I use whatever works. If Conventional Medicine works, I use it. If Natural or Alternative medicine works, I use it. If you don't believe a method works, without ever having tried it, well... whose fault is that? If you want evidence alternative methods work, try it yourself or go and do some research. Evidence does exist. However, not the kind of evidence demanded by drug companies and the FDA, who have set the bar high enough to keep out competition.

We Live in Interesting Times

Were you aware there are more out-patient visits to Alternative practitioners, today, than to orthodox hospitals? People are increasingly aware of the huge influence large corporations, bloated bureaucracies and unelected Czars exert over our lives. With the political-corporate 'revolving door' and influence-peddling corrupting politics, billionaire 'money-junkies' have a stranglehold on public policy. What is good for the wider population is of no consequence. Only what is good for their bottom line.

In thirty five years of looking, I've never seen or heard of a CURE from the 'modern' health system. There has been no end of headlines with 'Miraculous!', 'Life-Saving!', '50% Improvement!', 'Dramatic reduction! And 'Cancer Breakthroughs!' have been making the news every month for the last 60 years. It's a great way to convince you progress is being made and a cure is 'just around the corner'. Just send a few more dollars to your favourite 'Pink Ribbon' Cancer charity, (do you know how little actually goes on research?) and success is only a matter of time.

'We are fighting this together and we can win!' Poppycock. Tens of billions has been spent on public health and charitable funding, without a single cure for any disease. Yet they plead and plead for more donations, like professional street beggars. Playing on our emotions with heart-rending stories and emotive images of suffering and injured children. They are experts at manipulation. It's obscene to see young children whose hair has fallen out, being cynically used to make money for their poisoners.

We don't have a level playing field. Dr David William Kelley was written off by conventional medicine. He had tumours in his pancreas, liver and intestines. Tumours were protruding out from his stomach. He was in constant pain, his nervous system was being eaten into by the cancer and he had hypoglycaemia (prediabetes). Dr Kelley knew, in spite of the propaganda fed to the general public about success rates with certain treatments, there were very few people who survived the medical establishment's chemicals, surgical procedures and radiation treatments. He resolved to cure himself. Kelley had noticed eating some foods caused his tumour to expand a little and others caused it to reduce. Through much trial and error he worked out a diet for himself. One problem he found was the cancer 'die-off' made him very sick. He had to regulate the rate at which his tumours dissolved and find ways to eliminate dead tumour material. He also had to rebuild and regenerate his ravaged body.

Dr Kelley was a dentist and not a qualified medical Doctor. Nevertheless, other Doctors would send cancer patients to him, who he cured, using his pioneering nutritional approach. Kelley's fame spread until the medical authorities got to hear of him. Then, the harassment began until they eventually prevailed and shut him down. At one point Kelley wrote a small booklet about nutrition and cancer which ended up being banned in the U.S. This was shocking but shows the lengths to which the 'medical mafia' were prepared to go, to suppress alternative cancer cures. Kelley was made famous by the media, as the Doctor who killed superstar actor, Steve McQueen. The true story of what happened to McQueen has not been told. After being misdiagnosed for a year, McQueen was eventually treated for lung cancer by conventional medicine, and ended up at Kelley's door with only weeks left to live. Kelley was impressively making progress with McQueen, despite him still smoking and smuggling ice cream into his room, McQueen perished after an unauthorized cosmetic procedure and not because of the cancer. The media went after Kelley, all guns blazing. Instead of being lauded as a pioneer and hero, he was jailed, lost his licence and publicly crucified. Bitter and broken, Kelley quit. His methods suppressed for decades. Dr Nicholas Gonzalez (I highly recommend listening to some of his broadcasts and interviews), recently deceased, eventually resurrected his protocols.

The story of what happened to Dr Kelley has been repeated over and over again. I'm speaking mostly about the 'Land of the Free' but the same applies in most industrialized countries. In my opinion, the growth of alternatives cannot be stopped. In Switzerland, insurance companies are approving herbalism, acupuncture, homeopathy and such. Expect other countries to follow suit.

Will there be a new golden age of medicine, where true freedom of choice exists and serious alternatives are allowed to flourish? If the history of medicine in the last 100 years is any guide, not in my lifetime. All the more reason to learn how to cure yourself.

It Doesn't Make Sense

When you stop and think about it, it really doesn't make sense that, in this day and age, in one of the most developed countries in the world, with the best medical facilities and doctors on hand, the state of Public Health is so manifestly poor and getting worse. How could an affluent, forward thinking country like the U.S., have such high rates of diabetes, cancer, heart disease, depression and countless other disorders which simply did not exist a few decades ago? We constantly read of 'advancements', 'breakthroughs', 'progress' and 'wars', yet the health of the nation only deteriorates. There is a huge disconnect between what we are told and our day to day experience. Other nations, too, are sickening, as they adopt the western industrial lifestyle. The present medical model is unsustainable. The financial costs are unaffordable for third world countries and threaten to bankrupt first world nations. A diseased and desperate public have lost faith in our Doctors. You can hardly blame them. Consumers are crying out for cures. Yet, all we are offered are treatments. Treatments, which are expensive, unnecessary and hazardous to our health. Increasingly, we are asked to take them for the rest of our lives.

What else does not make sense? Today, we have a 1 in 3 chance of getting Cancer and a 1 in 2 chance of suffering heart disease. Disorders I never heard of as a child are global epidemics. How did that come about? It doesn't make sense to be undergoing heart by-pass operations, stents, removing gall bladders, appendix, tonsils, breasts or kidneys, when a few changes in lifestyle would prevent it. How many do not survive the trauma of surgery, suffer 'complications' for the rest of their lives or have to go back for more of the same, a few years later, because the underlying cause of their condition was never addressed? Do you know how many people die at the hands of Doctors? The numbers are staggering.

It makes no sense to saturate our food, air, water and environment with millions of tons of unnatural chemicals and heavy metals when the consequence is a poisoned planet. It makes no sense for us to allow a food system to operate which leaves us fat, malnourished, addicted and sickened. It makes no sense at all. Unless you are putting profits before people. Then it makes perfect sense.

Giant farms produce 'raw materials' for the Food Processing Industry, on an industrial scale. The Chemical Industry drenches these raw materials (soil, crops, animals and water) with a multitude of chemical contaminants. 'Big Food' takes the output, works it into different shapes, plasters it in sugar, fat, salt and fifty different chemicals with names no-one can understand or pronounce, puts it in fancy packaging, slaps a label with '100% Natural' on it and displays it on shelves. We then eat it. Does this make any sense? Not in biological terms it doesn't.

As stated previously, there is no food in a Supermarket. Just dead, deficient, toxic, artificial gloop, masquerading as food. So unnatural, animals won't touch it. Eating it produces a host of 'diseases of the fork', requiring the creation and maintenance of a vast health industry. Tremendous profits are realized at each link in the chain. Look at Cancer. In the U.S., treatment covering Stage I to Stage IV cancer generates income of between $350,000 to $1.4 million, per patient.

What else does not make sense? We are playing Russian roulette with drug medicine. Individual medicines may have been through clinical trials but combinations have not. Drug companies appear to be using the public as unwitting Guinea Pigs, paying only small fines (in comparison to the profits they make) if we are injured or die.

It makes no sense to spend a trillion dollars constructing an immense Security State to 'protect us from terrorism', while millions around the world die from our health system and we do nothing. It makes no sense to give Cancer patients chemotherapy when studies show the five-year survival rate for many cancers is 0 and the overall success rate barely 2%. Patients live 5x longer with NO treatment.

What DOES make sense is:

Proper Nutrition

Disease Prevention

Clean Food, Air And Water

Safer Healing Methods

"There aren't any", you may hear. Really? 80% of the world does not have modern medicine. Are we expected to believe not one person has been cured of chronic disease or cancer using natural or alternative means? Not one Arthritic? Not one heart disease patient? Not one diabetic? That such cases were 'spontaneous' or 'they didn't have the disease in the first place'?

Having witnessed people being cured using simple, safe, natural methods, I look at the efforts of today's Doctors, in disbelief. Anyone blessed with common sense knows most of us are sick because of what we are putting in our mouths. Yet medical schools teach perhaps one hour of nutrition. How can they not see the elephant in the room? We are suffering the consequences of excess calories, over-indulgence, toxicity and malnourishment. Eating when not hungry and eating for pleasure, not for health.

It is Not Your Fault

Do you feel lost? Helpless? Stuck in a rut? Do you blame yourself for your condition? For not doing anything about it? If you have been struggling with a health challenge and 'tried everything', yet your disease, or disorder, has failed to improve, you are in good company. Very few understand what needs to be done and even fewer do it. Those who find the motivation, make elemental mistakes. It is easy to blame yourself. However, it is not really your fault. You have just lacked important information.

For most conditions, it doesn't matter how sick you are. How many years you have suffered. What the modern Doctors have told you. Or how late in the day it is. There IS something you can do. Why are you waiting until your disorder or 'incurable' condition becomes intolerable before you act? STOP THIS THINKING IMMEDIATELY. Your disease or disorder is not going to spontaneously resolve. The longer you leave it, the more your disease will become entrenched and the harder it can be to recover.

Your medicine cabinet may be filled with prescription drugs, herbal supplements and a variety of 'Miracle' cures none of which helped you. So was mine. Your bookcase may be filled with health 'How-To' guides and psychiatric 'psychobabble', which made you a bore at the bar and dinner table but didn't cure you. Mine too. You may have spent months, years, or even decades, seeking a cure. Trying a variety of therapies, some of which gave partial benefit but none a complete cure. Likewise. I tried just about everything. Very few people are so fortunate to find that one simple remedy which might cure them. The 'Magic Bullet' or 'Quick Fix' we are so conditioned to expect.

Now you have the knowledge you need, the missing pieces of the jigsaw, you can try again. This time with the expectation of success!

What's So Bad About Treatments?

Treatments aren't so bad. They provide relief and allow us to continue to function. Aspects of the health system are truly impressive. The sophistication and innovation of medical equipment and 'tele-medicine' is a marvel. The health industry certainly deserves plaudits. What used to take days, or simply wasn't possible prior to the advancement of science, is now available to us, in many cases, instantly. For example, pregnancy tests. Hospitals are filled with gadgets galore, all serving a useful purpose. Although I must confess to needing a week to get over the trauma of an MRI scan. What a racket!

Yet, of what use is this sophistication when our disease or disorder is only maintained and doesn't improve? Of what use is Psychiatry if all the psychiatrist does is prescribe a sedative or a stimulant? For all our scientific genius, it is results that count and the statistics are grim. Millions are injured and die at the hands of Doctors and their treatments. Deaths so well hidden, the public is blind to the carnage and may even applaud it. Doctors, too, may be unaware of the scale of harm. A visitor to my home recently remarked he thanked the Oncologist, who administered the chemotherapy that killed his sister, 'for his efforts'. I don't think I could be as charitable. The oncologist almost certainly knew she would die from the treatment. In what way is he or she deserving of thanks?

According to a 2003 Australian study, '**The Contribution of Cytotoxic Chemotherapy to 5-year Survival in Adult Malignancies**', the 5yr survival rate of chemotherapy, overall, was just 2.1%. And this was taking the most positive view. Industry defenders do their best to downplay the study and its findings but there is clearly a serious problem with chemotherapy. For too many cancers it does not work at all and hastens the death of many patients. Yet they give the treatment, anyway. In fact Doctors are forced to give these treatments before allowing patients to try alternatives. Many physicians and scientists in other technologically advanced nations regard American cancer therapy as extraordinarily aggressive, using surgery, chemotherapy, and radiation therapy far more extensively than physicians and researchers abroad believe the evidence warrants. I should say at this point there are wide variations in treatments not only within the U.S. but between other nations.

[Note: There ARE a few Cancers for which chemotherapy has shown benefit and there may have been advances since the 2003 study was conducted. Please research this carefully. '**CANCERactive**' is a UK-based non-profit, Cancer Charity concerned solely with the provision of information about Cancer. Their web site is packed with the latest information.]

One motivating factor for Oncologists to use chemotherapy in the U.S. is they are allowed to administer chemo, to patients, in their offices, keeping most of the profit. They may see 15 patients per day. If they are receiving $10,000 per month from each patient, that's a powerful incentive to treat. Some oncologists are making millions of dollars annually. 600,000 people per year die from cancer in the U.S. 99% of those received conventional cancer treatment. Yet, isn't the charge alternative practitioners are only 'doing it for the money'? It's laughable.

So, tell me. If you inject toxic chemicals into someone's arteries, knowing there is a significant risk of death and knowing the success rate for a particular cancer is 0%, what do you call that? Is it even medicine? What would happen if someone who wasn't wearing a white coat administered this same treatment and the patient died? Wouldn't they go to jail? Why are natural healers, who have had success with cancer, brutalized, threatened or imprisoned, instead of celebrated? When you research how the American AMA and FDA persecuted Dr Max Gerson, Harry Hoxksey, Royal Raymond Rife, Rene Caisse, Dr Richard Schulze and many more, you will be shocked. The excellent documentary, 'How Healing Becomes a Crime' explains the health politics involved.

How many other treatments are like chemotherapy? If you knowingly prescribe a highly toxic poison to a patient who has no symptoms ('for prevention') and they die from the side effects, isn't this murder? How many HIV-positive patients would have lived had they not taken AZT? This drug made millions for the drug company, the gay community clamoured for it, yet their own documents show AZT was ineffective and a powerful poison. Tom Hanks didn't mention this in the AIDS-propaganda movie 'Philadelphia'. Gandhi called Modern Medicine 'Black Magic'. Quite.

Ask yourself...

- Is it really the case that, for so many of today's 'incurable' diseases, there is not a cure to be found, anywhere on this earth?

- Is Mother Nature so cruel, she would deny us the ability to heal?

- Is health as complicated as we've been conditioned to believe?

- Is it really the case only officially-sanctioned, qualified professionals can heal the sick or use the word 'Cure'?

- Do you believe we cannot heal ourselves?

My answer to all these questions is an emphatic "NO".

Some Doctors, the arrogant type (you may have met them) will bristle at such impertinence. "Patients healing themselves? Pah!" Doctors are certainly qualified. A talented bunch, better educated than I. They enter the medical profession in order to make a difference. Perhaps one, or both of their parents, was a physician. Or their career choice was entirely pragmatic... medicine is a rewarding and respected career.

Despite their undoubted abilities, Doctors are not 'gods' to be revered, as some of us (and some of them) believe. They have the same human weakness as the rest of us and are just as susceptible to control and influence. Possibly more so, since their egos convince them they would spot deception if they encountered it. Pharmaceutical companies and medical bodies understand this and direct a large amount of effort toward persuasion. Sophisticated marketing, manipulation of data, suppression of negative findings and recruitment of lead Doctors, encourages practicing GPs to prescribe medicine in a particular way. Do you really think it a coincidence the treatment you receive always involves a pharmaceutical drug?

What about all those studies 'proving' their interventions are beneficial? Peer-reviewed studies. Randomized-controlled trials. 'Double-blind' this and 'placebo' that. "Abracadabra!" industry magicians and their media handmaidens cry. The public applaud, little realizing most published studies are not worth the paper they are written on. That only 15% of 'scientific' medicine has ever been tested. Randomized Controlled Trials (RCTs) did not exist until relatively recently. The industry is not going to spend billions submitting 100 years of prior medical practice to RCTs. On April 2016, **The Lancet**, a highly respected British medical journal published an article stating:

'The case against science is straightforward: much of the scientific literature, perhaps half, may simply be untrue. Afflicted by studies with small sample sizes, tiny effects, invalid exploratory analyses, and flagrant conflicts of interest, together with an obsession for pursuing fashionable trends of dubious importance, **science has taken a turn towards darkness.**'

Pubmed is an online database housing thousands of research articles. In 2005 it published an article by John P. A. Ioannidis called '**Why Most Published Research Findings Are False**'. It is the most popular article ever published on Pubmed. The headline says it all. Over a 20 year period, it was found none of the 'breakthroughs' the media sensationally publicize (and they publish this stuff weekly) ever came to anything. Most research findings are unable to be replicated.

What does this mean? It means Science cannot be trusted. Results can be manipulated, research frameworks designed to achieve a desired outcome. Serial fraudsters consciously build their careers on fabricated data. Scientists pitch for, or try to hang on to funding, with slanted data. Studies are rigged for purposes of profit. Positive findings are published and negative findings buried. Billions in grant money is available to those who find FOR global warming, while NO money is forthcoming for those who find against it. Is it any surprise when scientists come up with the 'right' answer? How many media health campaigns are backed up by independent verifiable science? As far as I am aware no live virus has ever been found in an AIDS patient. What virus in history waits 10 years before it triggers symptoms? What kind of virus is racist, killing black Africans but very few white Caucasians? Millions of poverty-stricken and starving Africans, dying from diseases like malnutrition and infection, are instead reported as dying from AIDS. Why? Could it be because African Doctors are rewarded for reporting AIDS and not for reporting deaths from poverty. Instead of black Africa suffering because of exploitative western economic policies, they are now perceived as sexually promiscuous and spreading disease.

Lots of things depress our immune systems. Including gay men sniffing party drugs. The sores we observe in AIDS movies? Caused by Amyl Nitrate ('poppers') and its derivatives.

'Apart from causing localized damage to nasal membranes, poppers have been linked to anemia, strokes, heart, lung, and brain damage, arterial constriction, cardiovascular collapse, and, most tellingly, the blood de-oxygenation, thymus atrophy, and chronic depletion of T-cell ratio's associated with severe immune dysfunction.' - Ian Young

AZT, a powerful poison, causes the same symptoms as 'AIDS'. Like cancer victims who die from chemotherapy and are recorded as dying from the cancer, those who died due to AZT, were recorded as dying from 'AIDS'. Add these numbers to the African figures and you end up with 'millions' dying of AIDS. There is also the 'nocebo' effect. Convince someone they are going to die and they start to die. Yes, some people **are** dying but there are many things which depress the immune system. Whatever you may believe, and the AIDS theory is another one of society's unchallengeable truths, I strongly believe AIDS is just another racket. A trillion dollar racket. Why is there not one cure after so many years and so much money? Can you cure something which does not exist?

"AHAH! HEH HEH HEH HEH! So! You won't take warning, eh? All the worse for you... And now, my beauties - something with poison in it I think. With poison in it! But attractive to the eye!" - **The Wicked Witch of the West, in The Wizard of Oz**

It really isn't difficult to manipulate Doctors. Remember the 2009 'swine flu' which was going to 'kill millions' if we didn't get our vaccines? Doctors were outdoing each other to frighten the public.

- If WE can be driven by the mass media, medical journals, tainted studies, lead doctors and corporate-bought politicians, to believe in a bogus pandemic, so too can Doctors.

- If WE can be lured by 'inducements', such as promotions, kickbacks or seminars in the Bahamas, so too can Doctors.

- If WE are fearful of 'rocking the boat', being struck off, ostracized by our colleagues, stripped of research grants and perks, or left unable to pay off large debt, incurred acquiring our gold-plated educations, so too can Doctors.

It is difficult being a maverick when the bills have to be paid. Why make life difficult for yourself? The rewards for conforming are good, while the penalties for non- conformance can be severe. Because of this system of persuasion and coercion, you will rarely encounter a free-thinking, independent GP, able to dispense medicine in a way he sees fit. Not in the western medical model. You may believe there is nothing sinister in Doctors having to conform. How else can you deliver health-care to hundreds of millions of people, without some degree of control and standardization? If every Doctor adopted alternative methods, tailored for each individual, hospitals and surgeries would grind to a halt. Already under significant pressure, they would not have the time, or resources, to provide such a service, even if patients were prepared to alter their sickness-inducing lifestyles, which most are not. Yet, this is exactly what is needed, because industrialized, standardized medicine cannot cure chronic and degenerative disorders.

What Price Prevention?

If you have strong views about vaccines and are absolutely convinced of the safety of vaccines and in particular, mercury in vaccines, and believe anyone who disagrees is beyond the pale, it is perhaps better if you skip this section. For those who like a little scandal with their breakfast cereal, read on.

In 2011, the **US Supreme Court** ruled vaccines were 'unavoidably unsafe', giving vaccine-makers complete immunity from liability. Lawsuits were costing tens of millions and parents of children, damaged by vaccines, were lining up to sue. All vaccines are toxic. They have to be, to excite the immune system. When you look at vaccine ingredients, you can understand why they are considered 'unavoidably unsafe'. Highly toxic heavy metals, like aluminium and mercury, used as 'preservatives', cause the most concern. Not just for parents. In 2002 Members of Congress inserted a "hidden provision" into the **Homeland Security Bill** to prevent any lawsuits over the mercury based preservative Thimerosal. Also in 2002, The NY Times reported: 'The Bush administration asked a federal claims court today to seal documents relating to hundreds of claims that a mercury-based preservative in vaccines, Thimerosal, has caused autism and other neurological disorders in children.'

Official studies repeatedly find no connection between mercury in vaccines and autism (ASD). For those who accept official pronouncements, this is the last word on the matter. Except, it isn't. There are two main kinds of trials:

- Those conducted or sponsored by pharmaceutical companies.
- Those conducted by independent bodies or scientists.

The former found 'no evidence of harm', while the latter found the opposite. Similar to what happened with global warming scientists, who failed to support the official view, the latter had grants withdrawn or ended. A growing body of evidence has found connections between high rates of autism and mercury in vaccines. The corporate media never quote this research. Unless you go to 'dangerous' vaccine information sites, you hear only one side of the story.

'Scientific Review of Vaccine Safety Datalink Information June 7-8, 2000 Simpsonwood Retreat Center Norcross, Georgia'

Dr. Verstraeten, "…we have found statistically significant relationships between the exposure and outcomes" (*I have summarized what he found*)

At 2 months - an unspecified developmental delay.

At 3 months - Tics.

At 6 months - attention deficit disorder.

At 1, 3 and 6 months - language and speech delays.

At 1,3 and 6 months of age - **the entire category of neuro-developmental delays**, which includes all of these plus a number of other disorders."

Attendees at the meeting were clearly concerned. Dr. Johnson, "This association leads me to favor a recommendation that infants up to two years old not be immunized with Thimerosal containing vaccines if suitable alternative preparations are available."

Dr. Weil of the AAP, "The number of dose related relationships are linear and statistically significant. You can play with this all you want. They are linear. They are statistically significant."

In Denmark thimerosal was removed from vaccines in 1992. Data showed autism rates decreased as a result (Denmark keeps good records). However, you would not know that if you read medical journals or official statements. This crucial finding is either omitted from the literature or due to statistical manipulation, the opposite is shamelessly published.

We have been directed by corporate media to see 'anti-mercury' proponents as 'anti-vaccine'. This is shameful behaviour by the authorities. Seeking SAFER vaccines for children is the duty of every responsible parent. In the U.S. there has been a major increase in asthma in children. 10% of children now suffer from this disorder. How can such a staggering number be 'unavoidable' or remain unchallenged? Legitimate observational studies show a huge difference in asthma rates between vaccinated and unvaccinated children. When asked why asthma rates have climbed so steeply, officials feign ignorance, "We don't know". Like autism, the rise in asthma correlates with the increase in the vaccine schedule. "Correlation does not equal causation" is the usual glib response.

Official evasions and deflections don't impress parents of damaged children. If your child was normal before a vaccine and handicapped after, and nothing else changed, then it can be reasonably assumed the vaccine caused the handicap. A bit like waking up in the morning to find snow on the ground. You didn't see it snow, there is no scientific study proving it snowed. But there it is. Snow on the ground.

How trustworthy are official studies? Not much, it seems. CDC whistle-blower, Senior Scientist, Dr. William Thompson, 'openly admitted to taking part in altering scientific data at the **CDC (Centers for Disease Control)** to hide statistical links between vaccines and autism'. Apparently a large bin was placed in the middle of the room and relevant documents tossed into it. So much for the 'scientific method'. A new documentary about it called 'Vaxxed' was recently pulled from a New York Film Festival. This is a remarkable breach of freedom of speech. You can watch be-headings live on TV, all kinds of sadism and butchery but important information on vaccines? The truth does not fear investigation. A new documentary about it called 'Vaxxed' was recently pulled from a New York Film Festival. 'Trace Amounts' is another shedding light on this issue. Actor Robert de Niro, who has an autistic son, has called for the truth about vaccines and autism to be publicly investigated.

As someone who has suffered a lifetime of allergy and food sensitivity, and was painfully shy and nervous from an early age, I am somewhat distrusting of vaccines. One of the few memories I have of childhood, was my first summer with hayfever. Swollen, itchy eyes; runny, itchy nose, constant sneezing, and skin rashes whenever I played in the grass. I could no longer play in the local farmer's field, because straw bales would leave my eyes streaming. Allergy to grasses, one reason I am reluctant to return to Europe. During the pollen season I am confined to the house. Yet in the summers prior to receiving my shots, there was no problem.

As a parent, I have a responsibility to protect my children and want to hear both sides of an issue. So, when I see the media working so hard to silence and denigrate Dr Andrew Wakefield, it bothers me. Why are heart-broken parents, whose children were healthy before the vaccine and disabled after, excluded from the conversation? I have seen these medical and media tactics many times, not just with vaccines. Burning heretics is usually an indicator a cover-up is underway. Think Wikileaks, Tobacco, Edward Snowden, Asbestos, Fluoride, Vioxx, Thalidomide, Lead in gasoline and many more. Whistle-blowers aren't welcomed by the powerful. They are hounded and brought down.

Parents, who have gone through Vaccine Damage Courts, are clearly not responsible for whatever disease-inducing serums passed through a needle to their children. Now vaccine-makers been granted exemption from any liability, what incentive do they have to withdraw toxic preservatives?

If vaccines are effective and the number of vaccines we are asked to take is increasing, why is the nation's health deteriorating? 45% of the general population and 50% of children in the U.S. now suffer at least one chronic, 'incurable' health disorder. The extent of disease is shocking. We know diet is a significant factor; environmental toxicity another. Could vaccines be the third pillar of disease? Autism grabs the headlines but many other disorders are laid at the door of mercury and aluminium: Alzheimer's, Cancer, Attention Deficit Disorders, Bipolar Disorder, Asthma, Sudden Infant Death Syndrome, Arthritis, Food Allergies, Premature Puberty, and Infertility. Every Doctor knows vaccines cause disease, though they may deny it. Their patients tell them.

"My child was fine before his shots, now he keeps getting ear infections".

"I don't have one child who was not vaccinated who also has asthma or food allergies or Asperger's or autism or Crohn's or ulcerative colitis" - Toni Bark, M.D.

I am old enough to remember, during my childhood, none of my classmates had chronic disorders. Sickness was limited to chickenpox, measles and mumps, which were considered mildly harmful. Psychological disorders were rare, with the most severe confined to psychiatric hospitals. Autism among 40-80 year olds is rare. Since then Cancer has moved from 1 in 1000 to 1 in 2. Asthma to 1 in 10. Autism from 1 in 10,000 in 1983, to 1 in 88 in 2008 (in the State of New Jersey, it is 1 in 28). At the same time as Autism and Asthma rates accelerated, the vaccine schedule (and therefore amount of mercury) increased from 10 shots to 49.

The devastating effects, of mercury in medicine, have been understood for decades. 'Pink disease'(Acrodynia), named because infants hands and feet would turn red, plagued Europe, Australia and North America in the 20th century. The cause of Pink Disease? Mercury, (known as 'Calomel'). Teething powders containing mercury were declared safe and dispensed to infants. Up to 33% of those affected, died. Thousands more were irreparably damaged. Incidence of this disease halted only when mercury was withdrawn.

'**Ancestry of Pink Disease (Infantile Acrodynia) Identified as a Risk Factor for Autism Spectrum Disorders**'

http://www.ncbi.nlm.nih.gov/pmc/articles/PMC3173747/

In 2003, after a 3-year study called 'Mercury in Medicine', an investigative committee, chaired by U.S. Senator Dan Burton, whose grandchild received 9 shots in one day and is autistic, filed its report. I won't go into all its findings, of which there are many, but there is one correlation worth highlighting. Symptoms of Autism match symptoms of Mercury poisoning. One sentence in the report reads:

'In July 2000, it was estimated 8,000 children a day were being exposed to mercury in excess of Federal guidelines through their mandatory vaccines.'

A lead researcher, regarding mercury being used as a preservative in vaccines, said:

'There are other compounds that could be used as preservatives. And everything we know about childhood susceptibility, neurotoxicity of mercury at the fetus and at the infant level, points out that we should not have these fetuses and infants exposed to mercury. **There's no need of it in the vaccines.**'

After three years of Congressional Hearings on vaccines the **Subcommittee on Human Rights and Wellness of the Committee on Government** concludes:

"Thimerosal used as a preservative in vaccines is likely related to the autism epidemic. This epidemic in all probability may have been prevented or curtailed had the FDA not been asleep at the switch regarding the lack of safety data regarding injected Thimerosal and the sharp rise of infant exposure to this known neurotoxin. Our public health agencies' failure to act is indicative of institutional malfeasance for self-protection and misplaced protectionism of the pharmaceutical industry."

Mercury in vaccines isn't just 'in excess' of Federal guidelines. The WHO informs us there is NO maximum safe limit for mercury. The **Environmental Protection Agency (EPA)** say over 2 parts per billion in water is unsafe. Why then do vaccines contain 50,000 parts per billion? After 'realizing' the amount of mercury in the childhood vaccination schedule exceeded national and global safety limits, the **American Academy of Paediatrics (AAP)** and the **United States Public Health Service** called for the immediate removal of Thimerosal from all vaccines on July 7, 1999. Within 2 years, thimerosal was removed from the vaccine schedule. Except it wasn't. While most vaccine formulas were re-worked, influenza vaccines and Hepatitis B vaccines still contain mercury.

There is a diabolical dimension to the continued inclusion of mercury preservative in vaccines. If the owners of drug companies were to eliminate mercury completely, autism (and asthma) rates would plummet, just as they did with 'pink disease', exposing the lie mercury is not the cause of autism. It therefore becomes necessary to maintain current rates of autism. Such a thought seems shocking. Who would authorize such a thing? Well, the facts are the facts. Major marketing campaigns such as the H1N1 flu scare prioritized pregnant mothers and infants to receive mercury-containing vaccines. If, like me, you were baffled as to why infants were being given the hepatitis B vaccine, you now have an answer. Annual flu vaccines are routinely given to infants in the U.S. 'Accidental' mislabelling and 'using up old stock', are other reasons suggested for continued high autism rates.

'Thimerosal-Containing Hepatitis B Vaccination and the Risk for Diagnosed Specific Delays in Development in the United States'

http://www.ncbi.nlm.nih.gov/pmc/articles/PMC4215490/

The **Eli Lilly Material Safety Data Sheet (MSDS)** for Thimerosal (mercury) acknowledges exposure to Thimerosal in utero and in children can cause "mild to severe mental retardation and mild to severe gross motor impairment."(In other words, autism.)

'DPT Vaccine maker, **Sanofi Pasteur Inc.**, includes the following in their package insert (emphasis added):

"Adverse events reported during post-approval use of Tripedia vaccine include idiopathic thrombocytopenic purpura, **SIDS**, anaphylactic reaction, **cellulitis**, **autism**, convulsion/grand mal convulsion, encephalopathy, hypotonia, neuropathy, somnolence and apnea. Events were included in this list because of the seriousness or frequency of reporting."

Three of the above you may recognize. **Sudden Infant Death Syndrome (SIDS)**. Remember mothers being crucified by the media and jailed for 'murdering' their 'cot death' children? **Cellulitis** is of interest to some of my female guests. Caused by vaccines and not diet?

The credibility of official studies and statements is cast into serious doubt when looking at the Amish of North America, who do not vaccinate their children. Autism rates are 1 in 10,000. You don't see them dropping like flies because they have no protection, or being ravaged by plagues because they lack 'herd immunity'. They are very healthy. I just came across a media article about scientists examining Amish farm dust to find the specific particles which are protective against asthma. This attempt at pulling the Amish wool over our eyes is so farcical I fell off my chair. It isn't just the Amish. Françoise Berthoud, MD, a French paediatrician, studied rates of disease amongst vaccinated and unvaccinated populations of several countries and wrote a book about it called **'The Marvellous Health of Unvaccinated Children'**. If you use 'Dr Google' you can explore what he found (obvious from the title).

How devastated parents must feel, who, when it came to giving their children vaccines, weighed all the evidence, listened to their Doctors, received reassurance, then watched in horror as their children suffered retardation and disability. How concerned must parents be, looking at the shockingly high rates of retardation, to see States mandating child vaccinations? How worried must they be when schools refuse to enrol un-vaccinated children? This is forced medicalization of healthy people with substances known to cause serious side effects. How is this possible in a supposedly free society? An online post sums up parents' feelings.

"Mercury spilled on a school room floor is a toxic event: the school is shut down, the hazmat team called in, young people decontaminated, health screenings are done, and a major long term clean-up occurs. But, inject mercury into an infant and it's called a well-baby visit." - a mom, anonymous

A key factor when it comes to wider acceptance of vaccines and States ability to force vaccination, is fear. Fear campaigns are whipped up at regular intervals by the media until panicked parents and pregnant women run to Doctors' offices to roll up their sleeves. Fear suspends critical thinking. Media scares about this and that virus, over-hyped and always coming to nothing, appear fabricated to reinforce the need to vaccinate and engineer compliance. It is scandalous that pregnant mothers and young infants are prioritized to receive mercury-containing vaccines, during these media-driven flu scares ("cattle-drives"). At what point does the continued inclusion of mercury in any vaccine go from negligence, to collusion, to outright criminality?

According to the **CDC (Centers for Disease Control)** 35,000 per year die annually from influenza. Yet, there is no evidence for this. They base their numbers on cases of pneumonia, respiratory, and circulatory related deaths, without laboratory confirmation influenza was a cause. Because influenza is rarely an underlying cause of death, the CDC created the term 'influenza-**related**' death. One researcher calculated annual flu deaths to be around 250. During the H1N1 'Bird Flu' scare, in order to produce the required 'pandemic', the CDC directed that anyone with flu-like symptoms was to be reported as having 'Bird-Flu'. Many of these cases were elderly who suffer from chronic diseases. No laboratory confirmation was required. Of the handful who were lab tested none had H1N1. This cut no ice with the media who were clearly functioning as an arm of the pharma industry. Those thousands reported as contracting 'Bird flu'?

"No trials". "Unscientific". "Unproven".

Tamiflu was trumpeted as the great saviour of mankind. It was going to prevent a global pandemic set to wipe out millions. Never mind that it never underwent trials, the vaccine contained mercury preservative, and it was barely effective. You had to take it at the right time, would still get the flu, which might clear in 6.5 days instead of 7, and its side effects are worse than the flu itself. Tamiflu could never have prevented a pandemic, even if one existed. You know how this goes by now:

"No trials". "Unscientific". "Unproven".

Once the vaccine industry had made off with its billions in swag, having created a new global market for its products, 'bird flu' flapped its wings, flew off into the sunset and was never heard of again.

Another vaccine 'cover-up' involves anthrax vaccines given to hundreds of thousands of U.S. troops. **Gulf War Syndrome** is the name given to the set of symptoms experienced by military personnel involved in the Gulf War, and it includes cognitive problems, muscle pain, fatigue, diarrhea, and rashes. Adding insult to injury, the military called it an "emotional ailment" despite its measurable physical manifestations. The adjuvant (preservative) this time was not mercury but aluminum hydroxide. No other nation's troops suffered this 'syndrome'.

The issue is divisive. I once tried to discuss vaccination with my son, at the birth of my grandchild. All I asked was for him to look at the evidence for and against mercury in vaccines. He became angry. It had been hard-wired into him vaccines are safe and here I was, willing to leave his new-born unprotected. What kind of a scoundrel was I? This is typical of the indoctrinated. Today, his attitude toward official pronouncements is very different, having woken up to some of the realities of this world. Good for him. As an observer and parent of four children, the more I look into vaccines, the more troubled I become. There is far more evidence for the lack of safety of vaccines than the media and health bureaucrats would have us believe. If faced with a choice between a mild dose of flu, or autism, why would any parent vaccinate? The American public had been told mercury was out of vaccines. The truth was mercury remained in vaccines. How is it possible for an immature infant to receive 9 vaccines in one day? I don't need someone waving a study at me to understand this is utter madness. Considering the number of children damaged in the U.S. and to a lesser extent in other nations, the precautionary principle, pushed so hard when it comes to global warming, should have seen an immediate halt to the use of mercury in ALL vaccines. Instead, we are scratching around in Amish farm dust.

Another example of dubious treatments which, to Natural Healers, is positively medieval is the removal of women's breasts and/or ovaries, as a 'precaution against cancer'. With absolutely no symptoms whatsoever, only fear of the possibility of breast cancer, women are prepared to have their bodies mutilated. Can you envisage a young woman in her prime being given this advice, perhaps because a mother or sister, or both, died of breast cancer? Will her man really stand by her? Can she ever go to the beach again? Are there really no alternatives? How many women commit suicide after mastectomies? It happens.

This is a topical issue since Hollywood actress, Angelina Jolie, purportedly at high risk, ably assisted by the corporate mass media, recently encouraged women to have very expensive tests and their breasts removed, despite no symptoms of ill health whatsoever. This was a huge global 'human interest story' (marketing effort) and a sign of things to come with genetic testing. What happens if the public learn the risks were exaggerated? That the breast cancer test she relied on is unreliable or a negative finding can sometimes be a positive sign? That removing her breasts may still not save her? That even if the risks were accurately stated, strategies exist which can reduce risk substantially, or cure any cancer that develops?

Genetic susceptibility does not guarantee sickness. Gene expression can be changed. Will Angelina Jolie be re-presented to the world, with the same massive media exposure, making an unreserved apology to those women frightened into following her example? Unlikely. I do not know what you think of Angelina. My heart goes out to her. It certainly does not go out to calculating health corporation executives, signing up celebrities to foist ever more tests, 'wonder' drugs and treatments on the public, in order to sell genetic testing and milk every cent out of gene patents. This one at $4000 a pop.

Emma

Emma was still young when she discovered two lumps in her breast. After receiving medical advice, she underwent a double mastectomy and radiation. After her treatment, she went to see one of the top Alternative cancer specialists in the country, who provided her with a 40-page Cancer Recovery program. Emma, understandably, wanted to make sure she was clear of any remaining cancer. The specialist was sincere and knowledgeable but the document he gave her was an unmitigated disaster. A rambling, complex, political diatribe, so badly laid out it was almost impossible to read. I struggled through 12 pages before I put it down, appalled. No patient should be given such a document.

Cancer sufferers are under tremendous strain, even if they present as cool, calm and collected. They need simple, easy to follow, instructions. In Ayurveda, Emma is an 'Air' Type. Everything is going on 'up in the air'. These people live in their heads. They think too much. They need grounding, calming and soothing, not having fuel added to their mental fire. The specialist had thrown the healing kitchen sink at her, recommending 60 supplements, in addition to healing therapies. In his defence, the Cancer patients he sees have already undergone conventional treatment, so it is that much harder to bring about recovery. Emma's body had been weakened by radiation and surgery. Lymph nodes, which channel metabolic and other wastes away from the breast, were removed, for reasons which escape me.

Signing up for a '**Life After Cancer**' program or **Skype Health Coaching** provides much-needed focus and Emma is now benefiting from support, guidance and mentoring. No longer bouncing from therapy to therapy, skipping the parts of her program she felt overwhelmed by, or did not like. Emotional support has been vital. Emma has been through a terribly wounding ordeal. Grief for her lost breasts, fear the cancer may return (or is not completely eradicated), and the damage to her body caused by aggressive treatment, keeps her awake at night.

It is a testament to Emma's bright spirit and the love and support of those around her, she is holding up as well as she is.

The Fundamentals of Natural Healing

There are many books and guides on Natural Healing. Ayurveda, Thai Traditional Medicine, Traditional Chinese Medicine, Nature Cure and Tibetan Traditional Medicine. These systems generally have 5 stages and require you to:

- STOP doing whatever you are doing that is making you sick

- REVERSE whatever is making you sick

- Ensure all channels of elimination – kidneys, lungs, skin and colon are working optimally

- Clear your body, mind, emotions, energy system and 'spirit' of toxicity and blockages and bring them back into balance

- Provide the body with the raw materials it needs to heal.

There is an art to some of them but at their most basic, anyone can learn and apply them. What are 'toxins'? The **Nemours Foundation** explains:

"A toxin is a chemical or poison that is known to have harmful effects on the body. Toxins can come from food or water, from chemicals used to grow or prepare food, and even from the air we breathe. Our bodies process those toxins through organs like the liver and kidneys and eliminate them in the form of sweat, urine, and faeces."

Toxins include toxic by-products of digestion, metabolic waste, drugs, poisons, plastics, heavy metals, hormones, parasites, viruses, bacteria and fungi. Include toxic thoughts, physical, emotional, spiritual and energetic trauma and blockages. A colonic in your local spa is not going to eliminate or resolve them all, so how do you get rid of them? The blood is responsible for delivering nutrients to our cells, while the lymphatic system is responsible for eliminating cellular waste, including by-products of digestion. Nutrition IN. Waste OUT. If your colon, arteries, kidneys and lymph nodes are clogged with backed-up waste, (e.g. putrefaction in the colon) disease can arise. You are poisoning the organism. Waste matter that is not quickly cleared from cells can end up in the micro-capillaries of the joints, causing disorders such as arthritis. In Ayurveda, they call this waste matter 'Ama'. Once you have eliminated waste and cleared physical, psychological, emotional and spiritual blockages, you need adequate nutrients. Minerals, vitamins, enzymes, amino acids, antioxidants, fats and oils.

The above 5 stages form the core of any chronic, degenerative healing program and underpin all the major natural healing systems of the world. Where differences exist is in methods, quantities and kinds of supplements used. For instance, you can clear the body of waste matter by water fasting, colonics, juice fasting, raw food and vegetarian diets, exercise, steam therapy, liver, kidney and gall bladder flushes, skin brushing, massage and appropriate herbs and supplements. In addition, there are two 'live' components that are active within the human body. Bacteria and enzymes. Both of which, when properly balanced, have been shown to gobble up 'bad' bacteria, rogue cells and metabolic wastes.

Emotionally, it is commonly observed those who succumb to cancer, do so after a major traumatic event. Trauma depresses immune function. Natural, holistic, healing programs work to restore emotional balance. (The Emotional Layer in the 5 Layers of Healing).They do this by prescribing the 'blockbuster' drug, 'Nature'. Sitting by a lake, or in a peaceful forest glade, or on a quiet beach, or walking in the mountains. You can take it twice per day before or after meals. There is no black box warning, or side effects, apart from getting well.

The Great Lymphatic System

One way to look at how our body works is to consider what happens when we eat. We prepare our food in the kitchen, toss the food scraps in the waste disposal, where it ends up in the septic tank, then eat. What happens if the septic tank starts backing up into the house because the waste is no longer being broken down efficiently? We call someone to empty the tank. The same thing happens with our bodies. Our waste disposal system is the lymphatic system, which modern medicine pays less attention to than the blood. Blood makes up 1/3 of the fluid in our body and carries nutrients TO the cells. The lymphatic system, which is 3/4 of the fluid in your body, carries waste AWAY from the cells. Nutrition IN. Waste OUT. The 600 lymph nodes in the body are mini-septic tanks, heavily populated with immune cells, eager to get their teeth into virus, bacteria, fungus, pathogens and metabolic waste. Bacteria get a bad rep from modern medicine, due to the 'germ theory' of disease, which sees bacteria as the enemy. Prescribing antibiotics kills the bacteria in your lymphatic 'septic tank'. We know NOT to do this to the septic tank in our homes, so why do this to our bodies?

Most of us have compromised immune function and digestion due to the lack of live enzymes in our food (cooking and chlorine in water destroys them), while our gut bacteria (80% of which forms our immune system) is weakened or unbalanced by antibiotics in meat and farmed fish, and too readily given us by Doctors, indifferent to the effect on immune function and the body's defences. With gut bacteria compromised and unable to fulfil its protective role (along with a lack of live enzymes), Cancer and other diseases can take hold.

Once you understand the importance of the lymphatic system you can understand why surgeons removing lymph nodes is a mistake. Lymph nodes in the breast gobble up cellular wastes from breast tissue. Once those lymph nodes are removed, what then happens to cellular waste? Would the septic-tank company come to your house, disconnect the pipework and take your septic tank away? Of course not. They would empty it, or clean it and re-populate with waste-gobbling bacteria. Natural healing sees no need of surgical removal. It has techniques to break up congestion, clean the lymphatic system, mobilize wastes and clear blocked lymph nodes.

The Breath of Life

Another fundamental of natural healing is the use of oxygen. Mostly due to stress and lack of exercise, our lungs are frozen. We do not breathe adequately, utilizing only the top 1/3rd of our lungs. Neither taking in adequate oxygen, nor fully expelling carbon dioxide. This results in high carbon dioxide levels and low oxygenation to the cells.

Nobel Prize winner Otto Warburg found the prime cause of cancer is the replacement of the respiration of oxygen in normal body cells by fermentation of sugar, and the secret to preventing cancer was to maintain oxygenation within the cells. In other words, cancer thrives in a low oxygen environment (Anaerobic) and cannot survive in a high oxygen environment (Aerobic). Neither can viruses, fungi, bacteria and pathogens.

Oxygen is a great healer. Several very good books have been written about Ozone therapy, Hyperbaric Oxygen chambers and the therapeutic uses of hydrogen peroxide, which is H_2O_2 (hydrogen and oxygen). One such is called 'Flood Your Body With Oxygen' by Ed McCabe. In the book, Ed informs us, **'99% of disease cannot live in active oxygen'**. That being the case, let us celebrate a marvellously safe, cheap and effective way to cure yourself.

Increasing oxygen levels in the body is an integral part of most holistic programs, including ours. Breathing exercises (Pranayama) are fundamental to Yoga. If you are practicing yoga and not including breathing I suggest you change your yoga class. I teach four different breathing exercises, which are designed to flood body and brain with oxygen and 'prana' and remove stagnant air from the base of the lungs. If you are interested to know the names, these are the Bellows Breath (Bhastrika), the Skull Polishing Breath (Kapalabhati), alternate nostril breathing (Aniloma Viloma) and an exercise developed by a friend, Dr Paul Johnson, where you train the lungs to breath at 6 breaths per minute. Dr Johnson researched the breathing rate of monks, meditators, mystics and yoga practitioners, scientifically, to ascertain the optimum rate of breathing and 6 breaths per minute was shown to be the optimum. Sudarshan Kriya, from the Art of Living' program, is another breathing exercise I write about, later.

"If I had cancer, I would put a tube in my mouth from a juicer and leave the machine running"

Dr Richard Schulze

Curing a 'Great Great'

Dr Bernard Jensen was one of the 'great greats' in the natural healing field. A man who had written over 50 health books and treated royalty and nobles all over the world. He was versed in a wide variety of holistic health care disciplines including: nutrition, bowel care, hydrotherapy, fasting, reflexology, polarity, glandular balancing, sanatorium work, homeopathy, herbalism, diets, acupuncture, craniopathy and personology (a new one to me!). A man knighted for his work.

So how did Bernard end up, at 85 years of age, weighing 76lbs, on a morphine drip, dying of late-stage Prostate Cancer, metastasized to the bone? Perhaps because his lifestyle involved a lot of airline travel, long hours, restaurant food and disrupted sleep. Whatever the reason, he was given only days to live by conventional medicine. Until Dr Michael O'Brien was called in. Bernard Jensen wrote the book on bowels, yet had not had a bowel movement in 15 days due to the medicines he was given (orthodox medicines slow the transit time of waste through the bowels, causing putrefaction). Dr O'Brian realized, although Dr Jensen had fasted and tried various strategies to beat his cancer, he was lacking in two important elements, probiotics and enzymes. O'Brian gave Jensen oil enemas to move the bowels and large doses of probiotics and proteolytic enzymes. By the third week Bernard was conducting business over the phone and within 8 weeks, Jensen was declared Cancer-free and back to normal. It was a stunning turnaround and a dramatic demonstration of the ability of a non-conventional approach to cure.

That was not the end of the Bernard Jensen story. Shortly after reversing his cancer he had the misfortune to be involved in a road accident and became paralyzed from the waist down. Doctors said he would never recover. Once again, they were wrong. The same treatment was applied, with the same stunning result.

Within weeks Bernard was walking again.

Death by Medicine

Within the health system there are two major causes of death. Death by drugs, known as an Adverse Drug Event (ADE) and Iatrogenesis, which means 'Any unintended and untoward consequence of well-intended healthcare interventions.' When a Doctor tends to you, his intervention can induce either a beneficial or a harmful change. Most of us believe a Doctor's intervention is going to be beneficial. This may be true for acute and emergency conditions but for chronic degenerative disorders, it is not.

Let's take a look. The 3rd highest cause of death in America today, after heart disease and cancer, is death due to medical error. Between 2004 and 2006, in U.S. hospitals, it is calculated 238,337 deaths were preventable. In September 2013, The '**Journal of Patient Safety**' made the following shocking statement:

'...the true number of premature deaths associated with preventable harm to patients was estimated at more than 400,000 per year. Serious harm seems to be 10- to 20-fold more common than lethal harm.'

This was just within hospitals in America. If you accept these numbers, approximately 28 million people have died over the last 70 years from preventable causes, with 280 million seriously harmed. How many have died across the world?

There is more. The U.S. **FDA (Food and Drug Administration)** acknowledge 106,000 patients per year, die from taking the properly prescribed dose of pharmaceutical drugs. Read that again... the properly prescribed dose.

According to one Harvard study, systematic reviews of hospital charts found even properly prescribed drugs (aside from mis-prescribing, overdosing, or self-prescribing) cause about 1.9 million hospitalizations a year. Another 840,000 hospitalized patients are given drugs which cause serious adverse reactions for a total of 2.74 million serious adverse drug reactions. About 128,000 people die from drugs prescribed to them. This makes prescription drugs a major health risk, ranking 4th with stroke as a leading cause of death. The European Commission estimates adverse reactions from prescription drugs cause 200,000 deaths; so together, about 328,000 patients in the U.S. and Europe die from prescription drugs each year. The FDA does not acknowledge these facts.

This is just the tip of the iceberg. Excluded are those prescribed the wrong drug, those not reported at all, or those recorded as dying from some other cause. When chemotherapy kills a cancer patient, the death is recorded as being due to the cancer and not the chemo. Medical error is not included on death certificates or in rankings of cause of death. Doctors are embarrassed by failures and reluctant to report the mistakes of their colleagues. Even if you settle for this minimum figure, in the 70 years since WWII, approximately 30 million have died in the United States and Europe. Extrapolate that to cover the rest of the globe and we are talking tens of millions of deaths.

Isn't this a medical holocaust? So, where are the Spielberg movies, the Medical Holocaust Museums, the powerful political lobbies, the jailing of 'deniers', the billions in reparations, the solemn 'never again' vows, the constant media focus? When a plane crashes, killing hundreds of passengers, there are thorough investigations. The Aviation Industry learns from it and changes procedures, improves training, adopts stricter enforcement. In America, the equivalent of 4 Jumbo jets die each week from medical errors and what is the Medical community doing about it? Has anyone noted the silence? I have. 'Death by Medicine' or 'Death by Doctor' is hard to miss, when members of your own family have died.

A few years ago, my wife's elderly grandmother was feeling a little dizzy and out of sorts. As a precaution, my wife and I encouraged her to go to hospital. She refused, stating 'she would never come out again'. We insisted, so off she went. Grandma was dead within two weeks, of hospital-borne infection, her arms black and blue from clumsy, unsympathetic nurses trying to find veins. We naively thought hospitals were where you went to get well. Our ignorance killed her.

A White Coat Has Magical Powers

Doctors have an impressive ability to direct us and we unquestioningly obey. Public faith in the medical profession, although weakening in recent years, is still strong. We admire doctors' technical knowledge, cool professionalism and confidence. They ooze authority.

Is this faith justified, in the face of so much failure? Why do we so readily accept the diagnostic labels Doctors give our conditions, which lock us into narrow and inadequate treatments? Diagnosis is the foundation of modern medicine, yet we know most medical diagnosis is inaccurate. A Systematic review published in the British Medical Journal in July 2012 stated 40,500 patients, in America, die annually in Intensive Care Units because of misdiagnosis. That is the same as die from breast cancer.

Not so long ago doctors in America were recommending smoking as being 'Good for the Brain'. Today, they couldn't get away with such a claim. Or could they? Lead doctors (opinion-formers) seem quite happy to promote similar myths on behalf of their corporate sponsors. One example is:

"High Cholesterol causes or contributes to heart disease".

There has been no credible evidence presented this is true. In fact more people are reported by heart surgeons to die with LOW cholesterol than high. Industry is unlikely to backtrack on their claim while vast fortunes are being made from Statins. In fact, the threshold for 'high cholesterol' was lowered, to scoop up millions more customers and place them on these dangerous drugs.

What else is suspect about the high cholesterol theory? Dr Batmanghalidj, who wrote the book '**The Body's Many Cries for Water**' had this to say...

'It is surprising none of the frequently quoted and media-popularized doctors has reflected on the fact cholesterol levels are measured from blood taken from the veins, yet nowhere in medical literature is there a single case of cholesterol having caused obstruction of the veins. Venous blood moves far slower than arterial blood and thus would be more inclined to have cholesterol deposits if the assumption of "bad cholesterol" were accurate. This mistake by us in the medical community, and its capitalization by the pharmaceutical industry, has caused an on-going fraud against society.'

What about ADHD? They used to call children lazy, bored or mischievous. Now they are stamped as having a psychiatric disorder. 6 million children are being doped with Ritalin, in the U.S. There is little attempt to eliminate junk food and provide them with proper nutrition. No attempt to correct behaviour using good, old-fashioned discipline, either by parents or schools. No consideration given to the school environment which forces energetic youngsters to sit in fluorescent-lit pens and learn algebra. No actual evidence of a brain disorder. No attempt to remove 'excito-toxic' sugars, colours and flavourings from children's diet.

Parents and teachers accept the practice because, as we know, a white coat has magical powers. "No problem", the psychiatric magicians tell society. "Give your kids our chemical cosh" and "Hey Presto!" they are sedated. Parents are happy, they get to dodge responsibility for poor parenting. Their child isn't badly raised. He, or she, has a 'brain disorder'. Polar Bears are shown more compassion. In 1994 'Gus' the Central Park Zoo Polar Bear was seen obsessively swimming back and forth for 12 hours a day and placed on Prozac. An animal behavioural therapist determined Gus was bored silly. The zoo redesigned his habitat to be more interesting and Gus' swimming obsession tapered off.

Like politics, a week is a long time in medicine and we, all too quickly, forget the various scandals, scares and promises of 'breakthroughs' and 'advances' which are always 'just around the corner' yet come to nothing. Is our faith in orthodox Doctors justified? A serious dent in public confidence came about with the afore-mentioned 2009 H1N1 'Flu' pandemic, otherwise known as 'The Great Swine Flu Caper'. It might have succeeded in its goal of mass vaccinations, across the globe, if not for the efforts of independent commentators on the internet, exposing what they saw as 'a conspiracy by vaccine manufacturers to increase sales'. A German Magazine called the swine flu 'a total sham'. On the 3rd May 2016, The British Medical Journal reported...

'Key scientists advising the World Health Organization on planning for an influenza pandemic had done paid work for pharmaceutical firms that stood to gain from the guidance they were preparing. These conflicts of interest have never been publicly disclosed by WHO, and WHO has dismissed inquiries into its handling of the A/H1N1 pandemic as "conspiracy theories."'

BMJ http://dx.doi.org/10.1136/bmj.c2912 (Published 04 June 2010)

The WHO fuelled the fearmongering by claiming 7 million could die. National governments purchased billions of dollars' worth of vaccines, which were never used. I was pleasantly surprised by the public's resistance. Despite a massive PR and marketing effort to push the Tamiflu shot ("untested", "No trials", "unproven"), the public weren't convinced. After so many similar scares: SARS, Bird Flu, Swine Flu and the West Nile Virus (in each, the end of the world was nigh) there was a limit to which the public could be persuaded yet again to roll up their sleeves. The 2015 Ebola virus scare and 2016 Zika virus are simply iterations of the same push to shift product. The shenanigans of the vaccine industry raise a question. If the 'Swine Flu' pandemic was a fraud... and many believe it was... then what other frauds have, are, or are yet to be perpetrated?

"Doctors will have more lives to answer for in the next world than even we Generals."

Napoleon Bonaparte

P a g e | **150**

Crying Out For Change

When it comes to the state of our health system, the public is frustrated. I see it in the thousands of comments left on News sites, health sites, blogs, social media and from friends, over many years. The awakening of the public to the failings of modern medicine (and the system in general) is gathering pace. No longer are people prepared to unquestioningly accept. They are crying out for change.

- Crying out for an end to the idea we are a collection of independent organs, needing to be divided into separate medical specialties.

- Crying out for Doctors to address the underlying cause of disease, instead of managing symptoms.

- Crying out for Doctors to know the patient instead of relying on a few marginally-important data points.

- Crying out for Doctors to be trained in how to heal, how to prevent sickness, how to listen and how to educate, instead of receiving their on-going medical education from corporations, whose profits depend on compliant Doctors acting as drug-peddling representatives of the pharmaceutical industry.

- Crying out for health protection agencies to protect the public instead of acting as industry 'gatekeepers', keeping out competition and stifling advances.

- Crying out for Doctors to stop prescribing dangerous, barely effective, or completely useless drugs which require more drugs to manage the side effects of the first drugs, which trigger other conditions, requiring even more drugs... on and on... until we rattle when we walk and our livers and hearts give out from toxicity.

- Crying out for Doctors to inform patients of the true risks of their interventions and inform patients of safer, less costly alternatives, with demonstrably better prospects of curing a condition.

- Crying out for an end to over-medicalization, disease-mongering, unnecessary tests and bogus treatments, supported by bought physicians, manipulated studies and 'Junk Science'.

- Crying out for an end to drug companies 'inducing' Doctors to push their products. That so many Doctors are prepared to accept inducements (bribes) is a scandal.

- Crying out for Alternative practitioners to stop acting like conventional Doctors, substituting 'Magic Bullet' drugs with 'Magic Bullet' herbs.

- Crying out for the Alternative Industry to stop pushing fad treatments, useless supplements and bogus 'Miracle Cures!' so, like their conventional counterparts, they can drive BMWs instead of Ford Fiestas.

- Crying out for an end to a vicious medical monopoly which, while providing the illusion of choice, vilifies and persecutes authentic healers.

- Crying Out for an end to the patent system, which excludes natural compounds, leaving them 'untested' and unapproved, by the FDA.

- Crying out for truth and clarity in medicine. One year something is good for you. The next it is bad. There is so much confusion, people no longer know how to live healthily or heal themselves.

- Crying out for psychiatry to stop medicalizing normal human behaviour, so they can push ever more drugs and enrich drug companies

- Crying out for psychiatrists to stop conducting a war OF drugs on millions of our young. Developing infants don't need toxic 'chemical coshes'.

Ordering Pizza in a Chinese Restaurant

We've all experienced it. You aren't feeling well, you go to your Doctor and say,

"Doctor. I've read Garlic [or similar] is good for my condition."

It was a mistake to ask but never mind. If he's typical he will adopt his best headmasterly tone and reply with something like…

"I'm afraid there are no studies showing it works" [our old friend]

"If you take this it may interfere with your treatment"

"I wouldn't believe everything you read on the internet"

And just in case you weren't getting the message…

"If you wish to use alternatives I won't be able to treat you any more".

I'm not talking about all Doctors but you get the general idea. What you do not realize is the Doctor knows nothing about Garlic. It could be exactly what you need but the Doctor doesn't know that. They know nothing about herbs either. What little Doctors know about alternatives may have been mentioned in medical school but you can bet it won't be positive. Even if a few may know, they are unable to prescribe anything, due to the shackles of 'Standard Practice'. Doctors in the U.S. are incentivized to prescribe pharmaceuticals, via payments, targets and bonuses. A Doctor loses revenue if the public start to shift away from standard treatments.

The difficulty, for any Doctor who does take a sympathetic view, is they are going to be subject to intense pressure from their colleagues and medical associations. Even to the extent of being ostracized. A powerful reason not to break ranks. There is little incentive for Doctors to become better educated.

As the humorous Andrew Saul opines, asking a medical practitioner about Alternative Medicine is like going to a Chinese Restaurant and ordering Pizza. They aren't familiar with the ingredients, don't know how to prepare it, it isn't on the menu and you aren't going to get it.

Health Freedom

There is something wrong, don't you think, when people are forced to travel to other countries, perhaps at great expense, to cure their disorders? The Mexican Cancer clinics come to mind. Having been to India, Thailand and other countries and seen, studied and experienced safe, natural treatments that work, I am impressed by the health freedom these countries enjoy. In India, Ayurveda is government approved, as is Homeopathy and Gandhi's 'Nature Cure'. Tens of thousands of traditional healers, produced by the ancient 'guru' system, operate freely. Modern Ayurvedic Doctors are highly trained in both Western and Eastern Medicine. 20 years ago, the natural treatments I received in India were not available in the UK. Some of them are still not. Thank goodness for the internet. For all its faults, without it, we may have never heard of these safer alternatives.

Even with my knowledge and determination, it is difficult for me to find a skilled practitioner. Almost impossible to find one who will take on high risk patients. Some courageous healers operate under the radar but run the risk of prosecution for 'practicing medicine without a license'. People should have the right to choose the health-care treatments and providers they desire. Imagine my mother alive today with crippling Rheumatoid Arthritis, in a wheelchair and in constant pain. The Doctors can do nothing for her except pain management, using stronger and stronger drugs, with serious side effects. She cannot afford to travel abroad, as I did, seeking alternatives, even if she knew they existed (which she didn't). Her prospects are grim and she is going to die from the treatment (as happened). Now here I am, with two decades of knowledge and experience of natural healing methods. I know what can cure her, using safe methods and know her symptoms will be gone in as little as ten days. How do I know? Because I have witnessed it on many occasions and used these methods on myself, successfully. Terrific. I can go right ahead and put my mother on the same program. Or can I?

According to my understanding of the law, if I help my mother, I am 'practicing medicine without a licence'. Even if she did all the actual work and I limited my contribution to nutritional advice, it could still be argued I prescribed 'drugs' to her. How so? Lemons, Turmeric, Ginger, Garlic, Chilli, Vinegar, Cabbage, Celery, Carrot, Beetroot, etc., are 'food'. As long as these common items go into your Salad, Curry or Spaghetti Bolognese they remain 'food'. As soon as you use them for healing they transform magically into 'drugs' and drugs are the fiefdom of the Food & Drug Administration (the enforcement arm of the pharmaceutical companies). Thus, a fundamental human right, exercised for thousands of years, is criminalized.

In 2005 the FDA warned cherry growers in the U.S. to stop making health claims about cherries. The cherry industry had received funding from the **Dept. of Agriculture** to do just that, in order to increase sales. The FDA was not amused. The cherry growers decided to fight and the U.S. Supreme Court ruled in their favour, admonishing the FDA.

It appears that, as long as food is empty of all nutrients, it is "food" but if it has health-promoting nutrients it is considered a 'drug'. Not that any of this matters. If I felt I could save my mother, I would do so.

'The medical monopoly or medical trust, euphemistically called the American Medical Association, is not merely the meanest monopoly ever organized, but the most arrogant, dangerous and despotic organization which ever managed a free people in this or any other age. Any and all methods of healing the sick by means of safe, simple and natural remedies are sure to be assailed and denounced by the arrogant leaders of the AMA doctors' trust as fakes, frauds and humbugs. Every practitioner of the healing art who does not ally himself with the medical trust is denounced as a 'dangerous quack' and impostor by the predatory trust doctors. Every sanatorium who attempts to restore the sick to a state of health by natural means without resort to the knife or poisonous drugs, disease imparting serums, deadly toxins or vaccines, is at once pounced upon by these medical tyrants and fanatics, bitterly denounced, vilified and persecuted to the fullest extent.'

J.W Hodge, M.D.

Big Pharma

I was shocked, recently, when glancing at the list of side effects of a well-known skin ointment. One in particular stood out. DEATH. From using a skin cream?! Welcome to the world of Big Pharma. A group of gigantic pharmaceutical corporations that, since their inception, according to Peter Gotzsche, medical researcher and head of the Nordic Cochrane Center, meet the criteria of organized crime, according to U.S. law.

More than 70 percent of new drugs approved within the past 30 years originated from trees, sea creatures and other organisms. While most are completely safe in their natural form, they are less so in their synthetic form. There is no doubt some drugs are helpful but many are toxic. That's why we keep them out of the reach of our children.

Millions of patients content themselves with the relief pharmaceutical drugs provide. Especially when it comes to pain. Relief makes bothersome symptoms go away. However, think about what this actually means. Switching off the body's pain signal is like disabling a fire alarm going off in a building. The noise of the alarm is irritating, so we isolate the power and silence it. Later, another alarm may be triggered. We silence it again. Then, enjoying the silence, sit back as the building burns to the ground. In the same way, we suppress symptoms, allowing disease to progress.

If I were the CEO of a drug company, mandated by law to make a profit and exempt from any liability if people are harmed, would I be disappointed, or pleased, if a vaccine caused millions of new cases of asthma and allergies? Or anti-depressants triggered diabetes? Or the side effect of multiple vaccines was autism? Or radiation and chemo caused MORE cancer and a need for additional drugs? If my 'blockbuster' drug suppressed one symptom yet triggered two more, with all the profits that would bring, would I really ensure these drugs are safe? Or would I stay quiet, rake in billions in profits and just pay the fines? Judge for yourself...

'The European Commission has imposed record fines of 855.22 million euros (£534m; $753m) on eight pharmaceutical companies for operating secret market sharing and price fixing cartels in the supply of vitamins throughout the 1990s.

The heaviest penalty of 462 million euros was handed out to the Swiss based multinational Hoffman-La Roche. The investigators maintain the company was the chief instigator and was involved in all 12 cartels they uncovered.'

More examples:

1. **GlaxoSmithKline** (2012): Illegal promotion of drugs. Fined: $3 billion (largest fraud fine ever).

2. **Pfizer** (2009): Off-label promotion of COX-2 drugs including Bextra, Geodon, Lyrica and Zyvox, with "the intent to defraud or mislead" cost the pharma giant a loss of 90 percent of its 2008 income. Fined: $2.3 billion (then the largest fine of its kind).

3. **Eli Lilly** (2009): The maker of Zyprexa has had several court appearances over the anti-psychotic drug, which Lilly attempted to attract elderly populations suffering from dementia to try. The sales team were directed to disregard the law. Several lawsuits in various states resulted. Fined: $1.4 billion, $25 million, and $22.5 million (reduced from $2 billion for violating use of a product label approved by the FDA).

4. **Abbott** (2012): Abbott had no science to back up its target of the drug Depakote—an anticonvulsant—for use in treating elderly populations suffering from aggression and agitation related to dementia. But that did not stop the company from sending its sales reps into nursing homes. The company was also fined for promoting it as a treatment for schizophrenia although no scientific evidence existed to support that claim. Fined: $1.5 billion.

5. **Merck** (2011): The painkiller Vioxx was eventually pulled from the market in 2004 for its connection with an increased risk of heart attacks. But before then, Merck illegally promoted it as a treatment for rheumatoid arthritis despite any official approval. The company also reportedly made misleading statements about Vioxx's effect on heart health. Fined: $950 million.

6. **Allergan** (2010): Botox—the cosmetic toxin injected into the face to smooth out wrinkles and plump up lips—was misbranded by Allergan as a treatment for pain, headaches and cerebral palsy. The ruling also found the company paid doctors $1,500 to attend presentations on the drug's other uses in order to help the company push out its product. Fined: $600 million.

7. **AstraZeneca** (2010): After misleading doctors and patients over the safety of its antipsychotic drug, Seroquel, which included known risks of gaining weight and developing diabetes. The company continued to deny any wrongdoing. Fined: $520 million.

8. **Novartis** (2010): Between 2000 and 2001, Novartis used misbranded promotion of the drug Trileptal for treatment of neuropathic pain and bipolar disorder despite no approval for treating those conditions. Other Novartis drugs were also misbranded, including Diovan, Exforge, Tekturna, Zelnorm and Sandostatin. Fined: $422.5 million.

9. **GlaxoSmithKline** (2009): Between 1997 and 2004, the company was investigated for off-label promotion of Wellbutrin SR, an anti-depressant that had

been illegally prescribed for cases of bipolar disorder as a result of the company's marketing efforts. Fined: $400 million.

Fines a deterrent?

'Despite the large amount, $3 billion represents only a portion of what Glaxo made on the drugs. Avandia, for example, racked up $10.4 billion in sales, Paxil brought in $11.6 billion, and Wellbutrin sales were $5.9 billion during the years covered by the settlement, according to IMS Health, a data group that consults for drugmakers.'

Fancy a trip to Disneyland, Doc?

"GSK's sales force bribed physicians to prescribe GSK products using every imaginable form of high priced entertainment, from Hawaiian vacations to paying doctors millions of dollars to go on speaking tours to a European pheasant hunt to tickets to Madonna concerts, and this is just to name a few," according to Carmin M. Ortiz, the U.S. attorney in Massachusetts.

Everyone has their price

'Drug companies allegedly paid seven figures to three Harvard professors of psychiatry -- Joseph Biederman, Thomas Spencer, and Timothy Wilens -- who then went on to encourage diagnosing children with bipolar disorder and medicating them with antipsychotic drugs.'

Wondering where your Diabetes came from?

Johnson & Johnson to Pay More Than $2.2 Billion to Resolve Criminal and Civil Investigations

Allegations Include Off-label Marketing and Kickbacks to Doctors and Pharmacists

WASHINGTON - Global health care giant Johnson & Johnson (J&J) and its subsidiaries will pay more than $2.2 billion to resolve criminal and civil liability arising from allegations relating to the prescription drugs Risperdal, Invega and Natrecor, including promotion for uses not approved as safe and effective by the Food and Drug Administration (FDA) and payment of kickbacks to physicians and to the nation's largest long-term care pharmacy provider. The global resolution is one of the largest health care fraud settlements in U.S. history, including criminal fines and forfeiture totaling $485 million and civil settlements with the federal government and states totaling $1.72 billion.

"The conduct at issue in this case jeopardized the health and safety of patients and damaged the public trust," said Attorney General Eric Holder. "This

multibillion-dollar resolution demonstrates the Justice Department's firm commitment to preventing and combating all forms of health care fraud. And it proves our determination to hold accountable any corporation that breaks the law and enriches its bottom line at the expense of the American people."

Prosecutors accused Johnson & Johnson and Janssen of hiding the risks associated with Risperdal, which is approved to treat schizophrenia, bipolar disorder and behavior problems in teenagers and children with autism. Side effects can include weight gain, an increased risk of diabetes and, in older patients, increased risk of stroke.

The complaint also alleges that Janssen knew that patients taking Risperdal had an increased risk of developing diabetes, but nonetheless promoted Risperdal as "uncompromised by safety concerns (does not cause diabetes)." When Janssen received the initial results of studies indicating that Risperdal posed the same diabetes risk as other antipsychotics, the complaint alleges that the company retained outside consultants to re-analyze the study results and ultimately published articles stating that Risperdal was actually associated with a lower risk of developing diabetes.

https://www.justice.gov/opa/pr/johnson-johnson-pay-more-22-billion-resolve-criminal-and-civil-investigations

Regarding the case the **New York Times** and **Huffington Post** had this to say:

'Although it is encouraging to see the legal system to some degree catching up with drug company malfeasance, there are a number of problems with the criminal and civil cases brought by the Department of Justice against drug companies.

As in the case of the recent settlements with GSK, the company makes so much money from the drugs, they are little affected by paying out even $3 billion. Its stock rose significantly after the announcement.

Individuals within the companies, including the CEOs, rarely have to face individual charges or fines.

None of the money goes to the victims of the civil and criminal offenses, including the many children injured by the fraudulent off-label marketing of drugs like Risperdal and Paxil.'

On 25th Feb 2016, British newspaper, the **Daily Mail**, carried this headline… **'How Big Pharma greed is killing tens of thousands around the world'**. The article contained a number of damaging claims. The main points:

1. Too often patients are given useless – and sometimes harmful – drugs they do not need.

2. Drugs companies are developing medicines they can profit from, rather than those which are likely to be the most beneficial.

3. Commercial conflicts of interest are contributing to an 'epidemic of misinformed doctors and misinformed patients in the UK and beyond'

4. The NHS is 'over-treating' its patients and said the side effects of too much medicine is leading to countless deaths

5. The full trial data on statins – cholesterol-lowering drugs prescribed to millions - has never been published

6. One in three hospital admissions among the over-75s is a result of an adverse drug reaction

7. A 2014 report, by a panel of eminent scientists, concluded Tamiflu was no more effective than paracetamol

8. The medical director of **NHS (National Health Service)** England, Sir Bruce Keogh, admitted one in seven NHS treatments - including operations - are unnecessary and should not have been carried out on patients.

9. Former editor of the **New England Journal of Medicine**, Dr Marcia Angell, revealed, of the 667 new drugs approved by the FDA between 2000 and 2007, only 11 per cent were considered innovative or improvements on existing medications. Three quarters were essentially just copies of old ones

"It is simply no longer possible to believe much of the clinical research that is published, or to rely on the judgment of trusted physicians or authoritative medical guidelines. I take no pleasure in this conclusion, which I reached slowly and reluctantly over my two decades as an editor of The New England Journal of Medicine." - **Marcia Angell, MD**

There is much to be written about the history and behaviour of 'Big Pharma' and its collusion with politicians, consumer protection agencies and media ('Print that and we will withdraw our advertising dollars') but I will leave the last word to Robert Kennedy, who in March 1962 had this to say:

"New drugs present greater hazards as well as greater potential benefits than ever before—for they are widely used, they are often very potent, and they are promoted by aggressive sales campaigns that may tend to overstate their merits and fail to indicate the risks involved in their use. . . There is no way of measuring the needless suffering, the money innocently squandered, and the protraction of illnesses resulting from the use of such ineffective drugs."

"Drugs never have cured one single person having a disease of any nature. When it is asserted they have done so, it will be found on closer examination and argument that the person has recovered comparative health in spite of drugs and not through their influence."

Kiki Sidwa, N.D.

Why Alternative Medicine Does Not Work

I can't tell you how many different therapies and practitioners I've tried over the years. From Cranial Osteopathy to Reflexology, Re-birthing to Reiki, Acupuncture to Ayurveda, Past life regression to Biofeedback, herbs and supplements galore. My bookshelf is stuffed with 'How To' books. How to Cure Arthritis. How To Cure Cancer, How to Heal Your Inner Child. Oh… mustn't forget 'Scarf-Tying Magic' (Thanks Patti!) I was a sucker for every fad theory going. Finding a cure should have been easy. Yet, all that happened was I became confused. The more I learned, the more my mental bucket overflowed, the less able I was to make a decision. There are so many alternatives to choose from. Why did they not work for me and why have they not worked for millions of others who have tried them? It wasn't until I encountered Ayurveda and 'Nature Cure' the clouds parted and I finally figured out the answer.

Imagine having a healing toolbox, where each tool is a different therapy. There is the 'Nutrition' tool, the 'Exercise' tool, the 'Emotional Healing' tool, the 'Stress Reduction' tool, the 'Herbal Supplement' tool and so on. There are a tremendous number of tools available. How do you know which tool to reach for?

Imagine your house is on fire. The fire department turn up with a dozen hoses but only directs ONE hose on to the fire. It's not enough and your house burns to the ground. Now imagine firefighters directing all 12 hoses, at the same time. They have manifestly increased the odds of saving your home.

People rarely benefit from moving from one therapy to another, like a grasshopper on a leaf. You need to apply them ALL. At the SAME time. This was my error. Due to financial constraints and ignorance, I would try one. If it did not work, it was on to the next. If that did not work, it was on to the next… and the next… What I failed to realize was all these specialties are just small slices of a larger healing system. They rarely cure on their own because you need more than just one slice. Another crucial factor is you need to ensure the therapies you choose are addressing the **correct** Layer(s).

Welcome to THE KEY TO A CURE EVERYONE IS MISSING. Not just having the right tools for the job but knowing which to apply and when to apply them.

Why Supplements Don't Work

"Miracle Goji Berries!!

"Incredible Noni Juice!"

"Co-Enzyme Q10!"

"The Vitamin D3 Cure!"

Aren't you tired of supplements claiming to cure everything but don't work for you? Have you fallen for slick marketing? We all have. There are thousands of nutrients and phytochemicals existing in nature for Health Marketers to choose from. The sales potential is unlimited. Once they finish with individual nutrients, herbs, chemicals or vitamins, they can move on to combinations. The sky is the limit. The public hand over their money convinced this is the magic solution they need. The supplements industry is worth BILLIONS.

In a sense we are blessed. Thanks to legislation which protects the supplements industry, we have an embarrassment of riches whereby consumers can purchase virtually any herbal supplement they desire (except some which cure cancer), without the intervention of a qualified medical practitioner or pharmacist. We are free to 'self-medicate'. Bravo! I hear you say. But there is a catch (isn't there always?). This blessing may be a curse. Over the years, there has been an explosion of over the counter products (OTC) available to the consumer. You can find thousands of suppliers of this and that herb, with prices ranging from reasonable to outrageous. This is part and parcel of living in a capitalist system. Retailers constantly vie for your attention. Last year it was Vitamin D. Today, Cherry Juice. Tomorrow, B17. All backed up with miraculous claims to cure you of your ailments. The market is huge, profits spectacular, results pathetic.

What is the use of having thousands of different suppliers of Echinacea (an immune booster), if not one of them include Echinacea in the product!? As much as 90% of Echinacea products have no Echinacea in them at all. Don't believe me? Try it. Echinacea causes the tip of your tongue to tingle. Does this happen with the Echinacea you purchased from the health store? Such deceit is not limited to Echinacea. In a Press Release in February 2015, the New York Attorney General's Office informed the public they had asked major retailers Wal-Mart, Walgreens, Target and GNC to halt sales of certain herbal supplements. 79% of their herbal supplements were found to have no herbal DNA. The worst offender was Wal-Mart, with 96% of their supplements having no DNA from plants listed on their labels. Then there was the issue of contaminants within the products, not listed on the label. Such as rice, beans, wheat, houseplants and others. Yep.

That 'amazing' healing herb you are excited about was a dead house plant. Another example is honey. According to research by Food Safety News, up to 80% of honey sold in supermarkets and pharmacies have no trace of pollen. The small packages provided by restaurants and airlines have even less – 100%. The lack of pollen is due to ultra-filtering. Natural honey is heated intensely, filtered, then watered down.

How many of you have purchased OTC herbs and supplements and seen a difference in how you feel? Medicinal herbs in your typical health section are often formulated with little, or no, therapeutic agent in the product. If, by chance you improve, it has nothing to do with what is in the product but the power of your own belief. This is known as the 'Placebo Effect'. It is curious how, when a farmer makes healthy claims about cherries, the U.S. FDA goes after them, all guns blazing but when food giants strip away all that is health-promoting in our food and drench it with known carcinogens, not a word is said. Industry propaganda claiming organic food is no different to non-organic, is an attempt to mask the crime. In my view U.S. corporations are criminal enterprises. Food conglomerates make us sick, then pass us on to Health Corporations, run by the same sociopathic owners. These people bow down before only one God. Money.

Did you know herbs can trigger a Healing Crisis? The medical term for this is 'Herxheimer Reaction'. When your immune system is sufficiently strengthened by the herb, it starts to 'clean house', releasing toxins into circulation. This may cause you to feel a little unwell. A healing crisis is a sign your vitality is returning. Something to celebrate. You, not knowing this, may mistakenly believe the herb or supplement is making you sick. Opportunists, sniffing million-dollar awards, have used these healing crises to slap lawsuits on manufacturers, accusing them of harming patients. Manufacturers, due to the risk of litigation, have been forced to dilute their products to the point where they no longer trigger an effect, rendering them all but useless. When you purchase your herbal remedy and see no improvement, you conclude herbs (and natural healing) do not work.

What other reasons might there be why an herbal or 'Miracle Cure' won't work?

- Availability. Ayurvedic herbs, imported from countries like India, are blocked by Customs. This is purportedly to protect domestic markets.

- The herbs may have no active oils present, due to oxidation. Or their healing properties have been destroyed by processing.

- There may not be any herb in the product.

- Supplement companies have been taken over by 'Big Pharma', who have replaced 'live', organic, natural ingredients with 'dead', synthetic chemicals and crushed rocks. These are cheaper to manufacture and do not degrade. They also do nothing for you and may be toxic.

- Even when an active herb is present, the recommended dose isn't sufficient to bring about the intended outcome. You may need to take 5x the suggested dose before you experience an effect. Similarly, one person may weigh 120 lbs and require 2 tablets 2x daily, while another may weigh 240 lbs and require double that. Size matters.

- The individual is comparing herbal supplements to pharmaceuticals. When they don't experience a rapid enough response, they quit. Herbal remedies can take longer to work.

Were you aware of these factors? I certainly wasn't. There is one more factor, not yet mentioned. Perhaps the most important. You. I once encountered an overweight, middle-aged man, in a road-side café, sat in front of a plate of sausage, egg, bacon and fried bread. He was tucking into his meal, heartily, washing it down with a cold beer. I noticed some pills next to his plate. "For my heart", he said, flashing me a beaming smile. At the end of the meal, he lit up a satisfying cigarette. I was shocked this man would believe the drugs could protect him at the same time he was eating artery-clogging food, drinking and smoking. As if one negates the other. It does, I suppose. The food, alcohol and cigarettes were negating any benefit from the drugs.

This is the seductive appeal of Health Industry marketing. 'Do not worry. You can continue your disease-inducing lifestyle. Just take our pills.' A message sending you straight to the morgue. If you are smoking, drinking too much alcohol, eating garbage food and not exercising, why would you believe taking a single herb or supplement will undo all that harm?

Making An Herbal Tincture

Herbal supplements can work. Thousands of years of trial and error have shown us that. Modern medicine was founded on herbal medicine. Drug companies continually research natural compounds. But where to find quality supplements? Well, seek out an herbalist, who can formulate a remedy tailored specifically for you. Failing that, if you are the enterprising type, grow, harvest and prepare your own. You will be surprised how easy it is. The best outcomes occur when using wild-crafted herbs, prepared locally, picked at the right time and taken in the right dose.

At 6 am, during a full moon, you might observe me gathering bundles of a Thai herb called 'Luk Tai Bai' (Phyllanthus Amarus). 30 minutes after being picked, half of the herb will be bottled in grain alcohol and the remaining herb, already drying, will be made into a tea. In those 30 minutes I strip all the leaves and place them in a blender filled with 700 ml of 40% proof, grain alcohol. After blending for a few seconds the mixture is decanted into a sealable jar, then kept out of direct sunlight. It is necessary to stir or shake the mix daily. In 3 months it will be at its maximum potency and ready for use.

Why do I make my own herbal tinctures?

- Tinctures are the most potent form of herbal remedy.

- The quantity of herb used will be vastly greater than commercial products. They may use 10% herb and 90% alcohol. Mine are 60% herb and 40% alcohol.

- The quality of the herb is exceptional. Fresh, organic, picked by hand. No old leaves, twigs, fillers, chemical residues or 'stabilizers'.

- Its potency will be vastly superior to commercial products, having been picked when plant healing factors are at their peak (lunar gardening).

- It costs very little. There are no customs charges or shipping costs. You get more for less!

According to my Thai herbal, Phyllanthus Amarus is one of the most useful herbs known. Beneficial to the liver and kidneys, it is a wonderful daily tonic for diabetes and hypoglycaemia. It lowers high blood pressure, relieves stress, insomnia and anxiety. Is excellent for blood detoxification, gallstones, prostate and pancreatic disorders. A tonic for the stomach, and is frequently prescribed for fevers and back pain. Dried powder from leaves, twigs and roots can be taken as a tea, 3x daily. Making herbal remedies is easy. Try it with your local herbs.

Spooking The Horses

'Sudarshan Kriya' is an advanced yoga breathing exercise. One description says, 'This unique breathing technique eliminates stress, fatigue and negative emotions such as anger, frustration and depression, leaving you calm yet energized, focused yet relaxed.'

Benefits like this sounded great, so I was keen to give Sudarshan Kriya a go. Little did I know what I was letting myself in for. The exercise is practiced for 10 minutes each day as part of the **Art of Living** program (look it up). However, there is an extended session, lasting 30 minutes, which is particularly powerful.

How does it work? After a few loosening stretches, you sit on a chair, in a darkened, quiet room and start to breathe in and out, in a controlled, rhythmic fashion. A few slow breaths to start. Then medium pace, then fast.

Slow, Medium, Fast.

Slow, Medium, Fast.

Repeat for 30 minutes.

It is quite a workout. For the first 25 minutes I noticed little difference in how I was feeling, beyond the exertion. Then, during the last few minutes, as my lungs were working hard, I could feel the tips of my fingers and toes beginning to tingle and my body flooding with 'Prana'. Prana is the 'life force', or 'energetic' aspect of air, the Chinese call 'Chi' or 'Qi'. It is taken in through the breath and circulates to all cells. The tingling sensation moved up my limbs, until my whole body felt energised.

It is difficult to describe. I had never experienced anything quite like it. Few have. The 30-minute session completed, I lay down on my back in the Yoga 'Corpse Pose', as instructed, keeping absolutely still, eyes closed. A light blanket was put over me. All was quiet. After a few minutes, someone in the group started giggling and then all of us followed suit until everyone was cackling like hyenas. Laughter is infectious!

The first three times I completed this exercise, nothing really happened for me. On the fourth occasion, I decided to go for broke and put maximum effort into the breathing. The additional effort paid off. By the time I lay down, I felt super-charged with 'prana', my whole body tingling and vibrating, like a tuning-fork. After 10 minutes of laying completely still, mind lost somewhere in 'space', I heard a low moan emanating from within the room. The hairs on the back of my neck stood up. This was altogether different to the laughter of hyenas. The fearful moan increased in intensity, until it turned into a scream. A part of my mind was shocked to realize the person who was screaming was me! I was terrified.

What had created such terror? At the point my moan intensified into the scream, I became aware of a dark shape just above my upper chest, moving slowly toward my feet. The fear grew in intensity as the shape moved down my legs then exited via my toes. Suddenly, it was gone. The room was quiet as I looked at the others in shock and embarrassment. I must have seriously alarmed them. I asked the leaders of the group what happened?

"We do not try to interpret", came the unsatisfactory reply.

Whatever had been weighing so heavily on me was gone. I felt light on my feet and in my spirits. Dissatisfied with the answer (thinkers need to know) I determined to find out what it was. A possible answer came from a Sufi priest I met two years later on one of my jaunts abroad (Sufism is the mystical aspect of Islam).

"It was a Jinni", he declared.

Have you seen Aladdin and his Magic Lamp? Aladdin rubs the lamp and out pops a Genie. According to Arabic mythology, a Genie or 'Jinni' is a supernatural creature which can be good, bad or neutral. Akin to 'demons' in the Bible. Not a very nice thought learning my slim carcass had been occupied by a malevolent being. I wondered when and how such an entity could have entered me and then recalled an incident, four years previously. It was at the time I was 'in the pit'. That dark place, filled with despair, suicide and hopelessness, when my nervous system was completely 'burnt-out'. I had woken up from a fitful sleep and sensed a shape at the foot of the bed. Just as happened during the 'Sudarshan Kriya' exercise, the hairs on the back of my neck stood up. I remember watching, frozen with fear, as a dark, indistinct shape entered my body via my feet, moved up my legs, then stopped at my chest. I shrugged the incident off and went back to sleep, telling myself it was just a nightmare. But was it? During nightmares people wake up before the plane crashes, they are about to be murdered, or fall out of the sky when flying. Not this time. I was awake when the 'possession' took place.

What had this 'Jinnie' been up to for four years? Perhaps ensuring I stayed 'in the pit'. I did wonder, when I went through a later Christian conversion, whether the voice I heard in my mind, screaming at me not to go through with it, had been the 'Jinnie'. I rarely tell the story of this DIY exorcism, for obvious reasons. Western minds have been trained to dismiss such things. They are scornful and dismissive. Asians, on the other hand, who seem to love ghouls and ghosts, have no difficulty believing at all.

After this experience, my opinion of Christian retreats, revivals and spiritual workshops, changed. Previously, when my wife and I had attended evangelical revivals, we would observe people falling down, writhing on the floor, giggling or shrieking. At the time I thought they were all completely barmy. I still think some of them are. However, I am far less sceptical today about the existence of malevolent, paranormal beings. It would be nice if the genie could have granted me 3 wishes but this is real life, not Hollywood. Does my experience have any bearing on healing? Of course. There was no denying the lifting of my spirits.

Remarkable, unique, intense, rhythmic. Sudarshan Kriya was an amazing, 'supernatural', eye-opening experience. I think it is fair to say Sudarshan Kriya addresses the Spiritual Layer.

The Power of Positivity

The dictionary definition of a cynic is:

'A person who believes people are motivated purely by self-interest rather than acting for honourable or unselfish reasons.'

The dictionary definition of a sceptic is:

'A person inclined to question or doubt all accepted opinions.'

I have lost count of the number of people I have encountered who are cynical or sceptical about Alternative Healing. These types have little tolerance for techniques such as EFT.

"Tap my head while I am talking? Hahaha… You jest!"

Cynicism will block you from receiving the benefit of, what I have found to be, an extraordinary tool. There are justifiable reasons for someone not trying such a technique. You may not feel any empathy with the practitioner. It may be too expensive for you. However, if your reasons are due to fear, ignorance and/or unthinking prejudice, you might want to re-evaluate your beliefs. Cynicism and scepticism kept me on damaging anti-depressants for years, closing me off to therapies like EFT, which have proven to be invaluable. If I had remained a sceptic, I would never have been healed.

Where are you in your thinking? Are you a sceptic or cynic? Ask if your thinking is helping or hindering you? If it is hindering you, change. Is it possible to change? Yes!

My Destructive Humour

For 20 years, I served in the military, immersed in a culture of sarcasm and mocking humour. Men in the uniformed services are merciless when making fun of each other and I was a master of the art. Unfortunately, the sarcasm and cutting humour was not confined to barracks. Wives and girlfriends were often on the receiving end, whether at home or in front of others. When my wife Patti and I married, she had no idea what she was letting herself in for. Every time we met up with friends, she would be subjected to a barrage of barracks humour. She tried to take it in good spirit and be 'one of the lads' but eventually broke down in front of me.

"You are destroying my self-esteem", she said.

"Don't be daft. We are just having fun", I trotted out the lame justification.

After a few days of chewing it over in my mind, the penny dropped and I realized Patti was right. This was a new world to her and military humour can be cruel. I decided I would no longer use her as the butt of my humour. Having taken this decision, I was able to stand back. To be an observer rather than a participant. I began to notice the pain in the eyes of the wives and girlfriends of my friends, which caused me to view them in a new light. I lost respect for them. Patti had forced me to grow up. Anyone knowing me would be surprised at this transformation. When you have been behaving in a manner which is normal to you, you aren't really aware of any other way of being, so don't believe it is possible to change. I owe Patti a big thank you. She made me take a look at myself and what I saw I did not care for. Because of her I became a better person.

From Cynicism to Love

Growing up with a hypochondriac mother and an alcoholic father is going to have an effect on any young mind. In complete contrast to my emotional maturity, today, I was as cold as ice when it came to anyone being ill, emotionally or physically, when young. Years with a hypochondriac had drained me of sympathy. She would often faint in public, always managing to fall toward me. I would catch her, sometimes fantasizing about not doing so, convinced she was faking. Duodenal ulcer, hiatus hernia, heart problem, arthritis. Conversations always revolved around her health. Like all children, I wanted my mother to be normal. I resented the fact she wasn't and after one incident, cut her out of my life.

Around 8 years after doing so, I found myself going through a painful mid-life crisis and realized unresolved feelings toward my mother were part of my unhappiness. I resolved to face her, armed with a long list of complaints. When we met, my plan did not go well. It became clear my mother was not going to change. I had to decide whether to walk away and never come back, or find a way to accept her. Overcoming my disappointment, I acted with a maturity I had never shown before and made a vow.

"No matter what my mother says, from this day forward I am not going to react".

Mum lived two more years and died with a real, not imaginary, disease. Had there not been a reunion, I would have been racked with guilt and remorse. Instead I was at peace. My mother had not changed. I had. Instead of fighting for the kind of mother I wanted, I surrendered and accepted her, warts 'n all. Surrender brought forgiveness, tolerance and peace of mind. My heart opened and I was no longer emotionally cold when faced with those who were ill. In fact, the opposite happened. I became compassionate. The last two years of my life with my mother were a blessing.

"It's Too Difficult!"

How many times have you thought this? It is an undeniable fact most people, when asked to alter their lifestyle, even in a small way, find the idea unbearable. One reason Doctors don't bother and just hand out pills. I can give you an example from only a week ago. Steve is in his mid-50's. He came to me suffering from debilitating migraines and had been getting them every 2 to 3 days for the last 15 months. You could see he was fraying at the edges from lack of sleep. I asked him what he thought was causing them? He replied "Well. I drink every night and when I reach 3 beers, that's when the migraines start." I looked at him to see if he was serious. The blindingly obvious thing to do was stop drinking and see if it helps but that is not what Steve wanted to hear. He wanted some natural remedy that would end his migraines and allow him to keep drinking. Had I been a Doctor and he came to my surgery I would have planted my Size 9's firmly on his rear and booted him out the door.

People wring their hands at the thought they might have to give up the 'treat' which is killing them (that's the nature of addiction) or they have to do some work themselves. It is all too difficult or complicated. Rather, they search for another book, or practitioner, who tells them what they want to hear. It is easy to find a practitioner, or retailer, happy take their money. They have been doing that already and where has it got them? Is it really so difficult to make the effort? Think about it. How much time and energy did you expend on making yourself sick? Weeks? Months? Years? As a young man, having a good time, I believed I was indestructible. The pressure I was under built steadily, until, of all things, a spilt pot of paint tipped me over the edge into tension headaches, chronic anxiety, panic disorder, then suicidal thoughts. Reflecting on my lifestyle, it was hardly a surprise I broke down. How much time and effort did I expend wearing down my nervous system and thrashing my adrenals? Years. You may possibly have done the same. So why baulk at spending a few weeks reversing the damage? It isn't difficult. Only different.

Healing body, soul and mind is a fantastic learning experience. Many people who have come through serious illness and recovered, say their sickness was the best thing that ever happened to them. It forced them to look at themselves and alter their sickness-inducing lifestyle. Instead of being tired, depressed, self-absorbed and unhealthy, they become positive, outgoing, joyful and grateful for life. "That is okay for them but I don't have enough time", you may say. If you think you do not have the time then, before and after work, TURN OFF THE TV. Stay OFF your computer, tablet or smart phone, then see how much time you have. Or, take more extreme action and do as I felt compelled to. Resign my job, say goodbye to my loved ones and retire into the 'wilderness' to work on myself.

Once you decide you want to be cured, give it 100% and banish all doubts. With the right healing knowledge and sufficient motivation you can get well. The most difficult part is getting started. Then it becomes remarkably easy and you wonder why you hadn't started years before. What is most exciting... and I have seen it countless times... is that, once you start, you begin to feel better almost immediately, which then motivates you to continue!

What about poor old Steve? I haven't heard from him and doubt if I will. It is a fact of life that, for some people, changing their ways really IS too difficult.

Do You Want to Be Cured?

What a question. Of course everyone wants to be cured. Except, they don't. I can see the ones who are ready to die. Note the resignation in their faces. They have lived their lives, had their careers, seen their children grow up and leave home. They feel too old, too sick, too tired, or too depressed to summon the energy to fight. An end to sickness would be a relief. Death holds no fear. Some believe they don't deserve to live, convinced their illness is retribution for some past misdeed. Death the price they must pay for mistakes in life. Then there are the millions who are convinced their disorder is incurable. Persuaded by 'authority-figures' that nothing can be done. Those who derive some benefit from being sick, either financially (income coming from the State) or emotionally. They have been ill for so long they do not know who they would be without their disease. In a wheelchair, or on crutches, they receive attention and sympathy. Without it they are part of the anonymous crowd. It is difficult to shed disease which gives you some benefit. A part of you will sabotage your efforts.

Is this you? Have a good look at yourself and ask whether you truly wish to heal? Because if, deep down, you don't, then do not waste your time or the time of others. Time, better spent helping those who do wish to be healed. Stick with symptom-management.

I find this with alcoholics. When they come to see me, they are always adamant they wish to stop drinking. Yet, from experience, I know 9 out of 10 cannot be helped. Deep down, in their bootstraps, they do not really want to stop. Alcoholism has a vice-like grip on them. They need to reach rock-bottom before the message, 'you are killing yourself and harming your loved ones', finally sinks in. Only then can they be helped. I no longer help alcoholics. Organizations like Alcoholics Anonymous (AA) are better able to assist. It is too painful to put heart and soul into helping others, only to watch them self-destruct.

Stewart's Coronary Bypass

Stewart was a Type II diabetic, on Metformin. He had osteoarthritis in his hands and was a self-confessed alcoholic (at least he confessed to me). When sober, he was shrewd, intelligent and a pleasure to be with. When drunk, he was loud, lewd and obnoxious. A stereotypical Scotsman, some may say. There was only one way this man was heading with his health. Down. When Stewart came to me, he wanted to try a Homestay Detox. After 6 days of a 7 day detox, I saw him looking from the terrace, seaward, putting his glasses off and on, wearing a puzzled expression.

"That's odd. I can see more clearly without the glasses".

Stewart had done detoxes before but this was the first time his eyesight had improved. I put this down to the power of bitter herbs, particularly Bitter Gourd, which works wonders for diabetes.

"That is great news", I said. "Just keep taking the bitter and reduce the sweet. Stay off alcohol."

A couple of years later Stewart returned. He had not changed his ways, was still drinking heavily, his diet was poor and there was major tension in his life. His glasses were firmly back on his nose. Furthermore, tests had shown Stewart needed a triple-coronary bypass. He was understandably fearful of going under the knife. I explained to him about the Dean Ornish Heart Program and how it successfully reversed heart disease in 12-18 months, using diet, exercise, stress reduction and group support and he would be out of danger in only a month. The Ornish Heart Program has been scientifically validated. As Dr Ornish reports:

'These comprehensive lifestyle changes cause a 91% reduction in angina and significant improvements in myocardial perfusion and ventricular function after only 1 month.'

"Really?" said Stewart. "How come my Doctor never mentioned it to me?"

Good question. I suggested to Stewart, if it were me, I would go with the Ornish protocol but with a Ferrari upgrade. Here's the general idea. If you follow Dr Ornish' suggestions you will recover. He has proven it. However, what would happen if you 'turbo-charge' his program a little by adding:

Heart repair herbs, 5x daily

Contrast bathing/hydrotherapy

Massage

Castor oil packs over the heart

Fresh, raw juices, hourly, for 30 days

Wouldn't those 12 months come down to, say, 9... 6... 3... or less? Stewart liked the idea and opted for the 'fast-track' 30-day program. The knife still threatened. Plus, if he was going to go without his tipple, best to get it over and done with as quickly as possible. Alas, Stewart was an extremely restless man and found the program, "too restrictive". After six days he had had enough. He flew to the UK, underwent the bypass operation and spent the next year recuperating, counting his blessings he was still alive. Another heart patient with him, in intensive care, had died on the operating table. I met Stewart part-way through his recovery. He wasn't a happy man.

"I wish I had stuck with the program".

It is hard to comprehend the thinking behind why people do as Stewart did. When faced with a month of juicing, which is not unpleasant and brings almost immediate benefits, they would rather undergo major surgery and a long and difficult recovery. Perhaps they see the anaesthetic as somehow making it a pain-free experience. Or deep down do not have confidence nature can cure. Or they simply lack faith in themselves. Recent studies have shown heart-bypass surgery and the placement of stents to prop open arteries, is of little help in extending the lives of patients. Unsurprising since, if your pipework is corroded in one place, it will be corroding everywhere.

Are You Weak or Strong?

For many years, Dr Richard Schulze took on patients hospitals had sent home to die, and cured them. He was firm. If patients were not prepared to do as instructed he would not take them on. Dr Dean Ornish is similarly firm. If you are not prepared to stick to his program, you are out.

For many of us there is a kind of infant-like helplessness where we feel alone, isolated, weak and slaves to our addictions. Whether the internet, junk food, red wine, sticky buns, coffee or cigarettes. We don't believe we are capable of lifestyle changes and let's be honest, don't want to change. When someone says we must, we become agitated and resentful. This is the nature of addiction. When things seem to be going well, some of us self-sabotage. To return us to our uncomfortable 'comfort zone' or to flash our worn-out adrenals into life. The person in front of you is telling you to give up your 'treats'. The means you use to self-tranquillize. Don't they know how dependent you are? Where are you going to get your 'fix' if you are forced to stop? Our cravings are powerful. Just the thought of stopping weakens our resolve. Our inner voice whispers, "I can't do it". Like New Year Resolutions, our determination to make healthy changes lasts all of 5 minutes even when, at an intellectual level, we know we are slowly killing ourselves.

People love the information I share about diet, exercise, herbs, emotional healing and so on. They can't believe it is so simple. They have never heard this knowledge explained with the kind of clarity I provide. They are delighted to find someone to cut through the confusion. Then it hits them. They will have to make an effort. It involves sacrifices. I can tell the ones who will fail. Usually with such people I apologize, tell them I cannot help them and ease them out the door. Unlike Harry Potter, I'm not a magician. If you aren't serious about being cured, why waste my time? Practitioners like Schulze and Ornish do not need an undeserved reputation for failure, taking on those who know they won't stick with it. Stay with your mainstream Doctor. He or she is more than willing to give you what you want.

If you are feeling helpless and hopeless and struggling to stay on the healing path, DO NOT BE DISCOURAGED. Doubt is a dragon we all have to slay. As an addictive personality, I have had to slay many dragons over the years. Strength and success lie within each of us. When you see someone turned around from helplessness to hope as often as I have there really is something magical about it.

Staying on course sometimes requires a carrot and sometimes a stick. When I did my military service, heaven help you if you were a slacker. They soon licked you into shape. On one occasion I went through a 2-week Royal Marine leadership course. The emphasis was on physical exercise and boy, did they put me through the wringer. When I came out the other side, there was no way I could sit at home and be a couch potato. I HAD to go out and run, I was bursting with so much energy. You cannot expect seniors with arthritic joints, heart disease, or in a wheelchair, to start running up mountains and pounding pavements, being barked at by sadistic, shaven-headed Marines. There are less violent ways to get the blood and lymph moving. Yet there is a lesson here. If you are prepared to make the effort, though starting with baby steps, your transformation will amaze you!

The Right Support

Do those around you want you to be well? This seems a self-evident question. Of course they do. But do they? While natural and alternative therapies are becoming more widely accepted, anyone with a serious illness who decides to Fire Their Doctor and attempt them, can still find themselves pressured by loved ones, to abandon 'unproven' methods and follow the officially prescribed route.

One of the most common reasons people return to unhealthy patterns is the husband, boyfriend or significant other, objects. They do not want to eat 'rabbit food' (vegan or vegetarian diet), believe you are wasting your (or their) money. Or, deep down, fear you may change. Their instincts are correct. When you embark on a healing journey, more than just your diet may have to change. Your beliefs, values, lifestyle and relationships, which may be toxic and hindering recovery, need to be examined and, if necessary, changed. Healing from chronic disease can be simple and rapid, or it can require major transformation. The prospect of change can be frightening to those around you. They will fight to maintain things as they are. To keep you dependent. They may, at first, support you. Then, later, undermine your efforts. Keeping at you until you surrender and give them the 'old' you they are comfortable with. Is this your family, boss or partner? Find out. Then ask yourself. Who or what is more important? Your health or their insecurities? You can head off concerns by providing reassurance but the question remains. How far are you prepared to go to get well? What will you do if your relationship is a part of your problem? Are you prepared to leave? Throw out your husband, or 'significant other', as a last resort?

Long before alternative therapies became popular my mother told us about an alternative therapy she had tried. Applied Kinesiology. The practitioner told her she was sensitive to a range of foods. She, understandably, wanted to eliminate them from her diet. This meant two separate menus. Her husband wasn't happy. Money was tight back then. He was unaware of the importance of nutrition to healing and was convinced alternative medicine was 'mumbo-jumbo'. He complained until she abandoned her effort. Later, when she became very sick, he realized he might lose her and became wonderfully devoted, but the damage was done.

What about you? If you are trying to heal, do you have a supportive friend or relative? Someone who may have gone through it themselves and knows what is involved? A fellow sufferer, perhaps. Don't discount the Church. Spiritual power can move mountains and the Christian, Muslim or Buddhist family are the largest in the world. You do not have to be a believer for them to welcome and support you. You can seek support from Health Coaches, like me. Or find a 'buddy'. Contact me, online, or, if you need more structured support, join a retreat. There is no need to feel alone. Stress, depression and anxiety can drive us into isolation, sometimes to the point we will not leave our homes. Do not succumb to this. Realize that, while most people are preoccupied with their own problems, there are still good people out there. Be strong and keep your eye on the prize! Once others see you succeed they will no longer look at you as a burden but an inspiration.

Whether family, friends, or self-proclaimed experts; do not underestimate the ability of others to 'put a spanner in your works'. Having the right support can be the difference between success and failure.

Don't Run Before You Can Walk

Ellie was around 70 years old. Alzheimer's had taken hold and her family wanted to try and cure her, or at least halt its progression. Her step-daughter signed up for a 3-day juice fast and was asking questions throughout. This was unusual. A few days after she had completed the fast, I received a call.

"Mum doesn't look so good".

"Your mother? She is doing the program?" I asked, alarmed.

I rushed over, to find her mother lying on the sofa, cold and listless.

"No. No. No." I admonished. "She is too frail to be fasting. Make her some warm nourishing soup. Now!"

The reason for all the questioning became clear. In order to save money, the daughter had signed up to a detox program then fed back how to do it, to the rest of her family. This is where a little bit of knowledge can be dangerous. She had pumped me for information, soaking up everything I taught her but the crucial question of whether her mother should fast at all, never arose. Some types should NOT fast. If they are emaciated, they need building up not depleting. Strengthen them first and then try. Or, better yet, adopt a gentler cleansing program. When it comes to health, there is more than one way to skin a cat.

Fasting is perhaps the wrong label. Anyone juicing, is getting concentrated doses of vitamins and minerals, in liquid form. Far more than they could extract by chewing. Even if the digestive 'fire' is weak, liquids will still be assimilated and the body does not have to expend vital energy in breaking down solids. Energy is freed up to repair and heal. The concept of a vital force existing is called 'Vitalism'.

Caution must be exercised by anyone who is considering fasting. Your channels of elimination, lungs, liver, kidneys, colon and skin, must be working optimally before undertaking any detoxification program. You can become quite sick if you suddenly release a flood of toxins into your system. Experienced practitioners know what to do in such circumstances. The inexperienced do not.

Peter Seeks the Easy Way

When bar owner Peter came to see me he could barely squeeze out of his car. 54, grossly overweight, he had been burning the candle at both ends for years, and was now paying the price. Peter had serious health problems and was taking multiple medications. One step away from a coffin, Peter wanted to live a little longer.

"Wow. What a mess".

"Don't I know it", said Peter.

"How serious are you about getting healthy?"

"Very. I want a few more years with my daughters".

That was good enough for me.

"Ok", I said. "You cannot do this the quick way. You have to do this slowly."

What did I mean? Peter's body was 'filthy' from years of alcohol abuse, heavy smoking, no exercise, too many late nights and nutritionally-deficient, junk food. I doubt he had eaten a fresh vegetable in years. You could see it. Almost certainly his channels of elimination were congested. Constipation, fatty liver, enlarged prostate, fluid retention, psoriasis, high blood pressure, poor circulation, body odour, Statins (and other risky medicines), acidosis. Add parasites and fungal infection. Putting Peter on a juice fast would release a flood of toxins into his blood stream, driving up his blood pressure and overwhelming his channels of elimination. Peter could die. Before he undertook a program, Peter needed to ensure all these channels were clear and functioning optimally. I explained how he could do this. After listening, Peter was keen and hopeful. However, once he got home, he talked himself out of taking any action, wanting an easier way. Three months later Peter was dead.

There wasn't an easier way.

The Great Smile Challenge

When a Thai villager, with a smile that can light up the sky says, "foreigners think too much", it is a reminder of how much we in the West have given primacy to the mind. There is much to be learned from other peoples. I know because I've travelled to more than 50 countries. Lived amongst Indians, Chinese, Thais, Portuguese, Russians, Arabs and more. With few exceptions, whenever I travelled, the local people met me with brilliant, friendly smiles.

Who were the exceptions? Well, when showing Russian friends some photographs, one surprised me by asking, "Why are you showing your teeth?" He found it curious we show our teeth in public. Russians, in Russia, were also amused by efforts to make our pale, pasty bodies, brown. Such is the triumph of marketing. White-skinned populations equate being tanned with being healthy so try to make their skin brown. In contrast, brown-skinned peoples equate white skin with success, so avoid the sun, and plaster their faces with damaging skin-whitening chemicals and powders. The media and advertising world plant, then nourish, these beliefs. First create your market, then service it. Tens of millions are dissatisfied with their appearance, some strongly. It is a tragedy.

It is worth reflecting on just how much our perceptions of ourselves have been shaped by corporations. Their goal is, in every aspect of our being, to make us dissatisfied, in order to sell us the solution. Be it cosmetics, 'diet' products, suntan lotion, sneakers and so on. Liberating yourself from false conditioning is absolutely necessary, if you are ever to be confident in yourself and free.

For all its faults, religion has a better model. Isn't it better to be a seen as perfect in God's eyes, made 'in the image of God', than to be convinced by an advertising company you are too fat, too white, too black, your teeth too yellow or misshapen, your nose too big, breasts too small? Why go through life believing these things about yourself? Here's my rather basic suggestion. Stick two fingers up at these deceivers and scoundrels and STAND TALL. You ARE perfect. Nature does not make mistakes. What kind of a boring world would it be if we all looked like Brad Pitt and Angelina Jolie? I once suggested to an artist friend I might have a little nip and tuck. Remove the skin under my eyes or from around my neck which, in my advancing years, looks rather like a freshly plucked chicken. I look my age. Unacceptable in this latest 'anti-aging' fad. To her credit, my friend gave me a withering look which said, if you change a thing, I'll kill you! So I accepted my outer coating wasn't going to get any younger and surrendered to the fact my life experiences, good and bad, are etched permanently onto my face and chicken-skin neck.

Coming back to smiling. In Moscow and St. Petersburg I rarely saw anyone smile in the street, yet, experienced genuine warmth inside apartments. In India, Cambodia, Laos, Vietnam and Thailand, the villagers smile instantly and invite me into their homes for 'chai' (tea), or food. In India, this impressed me so much I decided to conduct an experiment. For a two week period I would smile at every traveller I met. It was revealing. European and American travellers were stone-faced. Many would not look me in the eye. They seemed pre-occupied, troubled and almost alarmed when I smiled at them. Why is this 'weirdo' grinning at me?! One or two returned the smile, in surprise and pleasure. We have forgotten how to smile at each other. To relax and greet each other as fellow inhabitants of this beautiful planet. To experience the joy of new encounters and new friends. It's a little sad, don't you think?

There is a fascinating video online showing laughter spreading on a New York subway. You may have seen it. It did not take much to have everyone laughing. Try it next time you are out and about. Or if you can't bring yourself to chuckle, smile at others and see the reaction you get. Call it 'The Great Smile Challenge'. Email me and share your experience.

EFT + NLP

EFT (Emotional Freedom Technique) is a very simple method for dissolving emotional issues and curing addictions. Using the tips of your fingers, you tap on certain energy meridians, in a particular sequence, while focussing on whatever trauma, addiction or fear you wish to dissolve. EFT has been described as 'Acupuncture without the needles'.

NLP (Neuro-Linguistic Programming) is claimed to be a way of providing shortcuts to success in life, by altering our thinking and beliefs. To look at what thoughts hold us back and what thoughts advance us. The word 'programming' sounds a bit creepy but it is not at all. Therapists identify the negative language we use and encourage us to replace it with positive statements. How do the two work together? If I am scared of spiders and say to myself (the conscious mind), "I am NOT scared of spiders", it does not work because my subconscious mind has "I AM scared of spiders" written to its internal hard drive. This is how we can be 'in two minds'. It does not matter what you tell yourself, consciously. You need to be able to change the belief embedded in your unconscious. This is where EFT and NLP work together beautifully. EFT, for reasons I have yet to understand but do not really care just as long as it works, dissolves the emotions attached to beliefs, reducing their power to the point a new belief can be inserted into the unconscious. E.g. Delete 'I am scared of spiders' and insert 'Spiders don't bother me'.

In my experience, EFT has around a 70% success rate. This is way in excess of anything Psychiatry achieves and without the need for medication. It costs very little and results can be seen within minutes.

"It's Only Two a Day!"

I could hear the gasping of the over-laden 'tuk-tuk' (motorbike taxi) as it climbed the hill and pulled up in front of the gate. From my rear garden, I observed three ladies disembark. Angela was young and heavy. Susan, middle aged, and attractive. Erin, elderly and obese. They had heard of me and wanted to discuss their various health issues. Angela had been an athlete when she was younger and a very good one, representing her country, in gymnastics, until a family tragedy. Then came over-eating, weight gain and depression. For 12 years Doctors and psychiatrists, unable to figure out what was wrong with her, only dispensed drugs. Angela was tired of it all. Susan was different. She didn't look unwell and it turns out, wasn't. Unless trying to stay young is a sickness. No. Susan was on a mission. Looking for anything that would help her sick mother, suffering from Alzheimer's. Erin was seriously unwell. God knows how she managed to draw breath. Cancer, heart disease, obesity and a variety of other conditions. Erin had spent years in and out of hospitals, undergoing multiple operations.

Drinks were served, pleasantries exchanged. I started to share some of my knowledge. It quickly became apparent Erin was very clued-up on the alternative medical scene. There is very little she didn't know and hadn't tried and she became animated as she confirmed my opinions and offered some of her own. It was all hugely supportive. The meeting was going swimmingly, until Erin suddenly reached into her bag, pulled out a cigarette and lit up.

"Gasp!"

No. This was not Erin gasping for the cigarette; it was the simultaneous sound of the rest of us expressing shock. I'm sure you are wondering the same thing we did. How can a person, who is so seriously ill, has cheated death so often, with such a tremendous amount of knowledge and experience, smoke? There was a huge contradiction at work here. I explained to Erin I could not help her if she smoked. Nicotine is a vaso-constrictor. It restricts blood flow, the opposite of what we try to achieve.

"But it's only two a day!" she cried.

"I'm sorry. Those are my rules".

That was the last I saw of Erin.

Psychiatry - A Dark Art

Psychiatry merits a book in itself. I cannot do the topic justice here so will settle for giving you a taster. Psychiatry may wrap itself in medical clothes but it lacks any credible science. Where do they get all these disorders from? An ever-increasing list of human behaviours is voted on, with a show of hands, by members of the American Psychiatric Association, most of whom have ties to pharmaceutical companies, and labelled 'disorders'. The result? The mass poisoning of society with toxic chemistry.

Language in Medicine is interesting. Take the word 'Sedative' or 'Sedate'. It's a nice word. Comforting, soothing, positive, appealing. Your mind is out of control, filled with dark, oppressive thoughts, exercising a form of tyranny over you, so you cannot sleep, function, relate to others, and your psychiatrist says "Here's a sedative to calm you down and help you sleep". Who wouldn't be seduced by such language? Yet, what if the Psychiatrist said, "I have a toxic poison, which will make you docile, destroys your sexual function, causes permanent brain changes, turns you into a life-long addict, causes the very symptoms you are trying to relieve, will give you diabetes, triggers suicide and will block you from reaching higher states of consciousness". You would be out of the door in a hurry.

The 'Bible' of Psychiatry is called the "Diagnostic and Statistical Manual" (DSM). The latest version, DSM-5, is basically a billing system for insurance companies and governments. Psychiatry, in my opinion, is appropriate for only a few seriously disturbed individuals. Not what we see today, the wholesale drugging of the masses. Psychiatry has a history which is medieval in its barbarity and cruelty. While some of the more gruesome practices have ended, running electricity through someone's body and administering fluoride-based 'chemical coshes', to adults and infants alike, is State-sponsored violence upon the individual. Hippocrates instruction to 'first do no harm' is clearly absent. Side effects of anti-depressants include permanent brain changes, sexual dysfunction and diabetes.

Approximately 1 in 4 adult Americans have been diagnosed with a mental disorder in the last 12 months. Diagnoses include major depression, bipolar disorder, schizophrenia and anxiety disorders, eating disorders, attention deficit disorder/attention deficit hyperactivity disorder (ADD/ADHD) and addiction. Worldwide, incidence rates range from a staggering 26% of the population in America, to 4% in China. That statistic, alone, should tell you something is seriously amiss in America. What is behind this incredible rise? Are there really so many 'Mad Dads' (as someone once called me) 'Crazy Mums' and 'Barmy Kids' out there? Critics say most psychiatric disorders are sheer inventions. Disease-mongering, creating the illusion of widespread mental illness. The normal vagaries of life, labelled a 'disorder', for corporate profit and population control. When 2-year olds are being diagnosed with 'Bipolar Disorder' and drugged, you are not looking at medicine but evil. Billions of dollars can be made from the sale of one drug... even a bad drug... if you have the right marketing campaign. Psychiatric drugs generate $billions.

Alternative medicine is castigated and dismissed for 'not having any science to support it'. Psychiatry has less yet is fully supported by government. Where is the test for a chemical imbalance of the brain? I have never seen or been offered one. Yet the industry still peddles this psychiatric equivalent of, "It's Genetic". Emotional trauma can be upsetting and some people need support. This used to be provided by family, community and the local priest.

The vast majority of mental health problems are due to poverty, poor parenting, war, toxic environment, lack of education, the mass media pouring negativity, conflict and fear into our minds, and nutritional deficiency. Stress is a major cause of physical and mental illness. The term 'toxic stress' has been coined to describe it. This Harvard article explains:

'When toxic stress response occurs continually, or is triggered by multiple sources, it can have a cumulative toll on an individual's physical and mental health—for a lifetime. The more adverse experiences in childhood, the greater the likelihood of developmental delays and later health problems, including heart disease, diabetes, substance abuse, and depression.'

If I am experiencing stress because I have lost my job or am going through a painful divorce, or the media are instilling fear in me, the way to relieve that stress is to provide me with employment, repair the relationship and switch off the TV. Poisoning my body and brain with toxic chemicals, does nothing to resolve underlying cause. A disturbed child does not need fluoride, or Class II narcotics, like Ritalin. He or she needs a secure, safe, supportive environment. Young brains ARE subjected to an increasing number of developmental toxins, such as glutamine, aspartame, fluoride, lead, arsenic, pcb's, toluene, vaccine ingredients and more. Additionally, the young are being turned into uncontrollable monsters by subversive messages in cartoons and on TV. They are trained to defy parents and demand ice cream, burgers, coke and sweets. Teens are turned into sexualized sluts and knuckle-dragging thugs, by a corrupt music industry, whose intent appears to be the degradation of society. Is the remedy for this really to imbibe a poison?

The steady diet of 'Zombie' movies from Hollywood is a perverse celebration of man being separated from the Divine. Millions are kept trapped in a waking sleep, their senses deliberately stupefied. No highs, no lows. You function but are dead to any feeling. Try to end dependence on chemicals and your anxiety worsens and suicidal thoughts arise. The name Hollywood is interesting. Did you know the ancient English druids cast spells using a 'magic wand'? The wand was made from the wood of the holly tree. Holly... wood... Hollywood. It certainly looks to me like Hollywood 'casts spells'. Not only Hollywood. The music industry, TV, Newspapers and the internet. All working in lock-step, capturing our attention, telling us what to think, who to hate, what to wear and who to copy. Are these 'spell-binders' promoting peace of mind, love, compassion, tolerance, forgiveness, selflessness, harmony, social cohesion, happiness and cultural respect? Or are they promoting fear, terror, violence, selfishness, materialism, hatred for each other, warmongering, social engineering, instant gratification and 'anything goes'? Do you think you are immune to it? Is this REALLY what you want to be feeding your mind and the minds of your children?

It has been my observation many Psychiatrists are themselves troubled. Choosing psychiatry to work out their inner demons and not succeeding. Hardly surprising. If they cannot fix patients, only stupefy them, how can they fix themselves? Drug-peddling works. The pharmaceutical industry makes money. The medical and psychiatric professions make money. Their political partners-in-crime make money. Insurers make money. The only one left out of the party is the patient. When Peter Gotzsche, described the largest pharmaceutical companies as "organized crime", he might have been looking at psychiatry. In my opinion, Psychiatry is not a Science, it's a Dark Art.

When detoxing your body, take care to also detox your mind, of the psychological and spiritual poisons implanted in you. Turn off the TV, stop watching Hollywood movies and cartoons. Stay away from porn sites. Don't allow these agencies to capture your mind or the mind of your children. Feed your mind the positive qualities listed.

The Power of Miracles

'MIRACLE CURES!' Don't you just love them? Available online, for a one-time-only bargain price, guaranteed to cure every ailment. The well-intentioned, alongside 'Snake Oil' salesmen, draw us in with fantastical claims and testimonials of miracle cures, selling us DVDs, books and products, which invariably fail. They may have worked for the seller but they did not work for us.

The King of miracles was Jesus. If we could only touch the hem of his garment, we would all be healed. As a child I was an angelic choirboy. Later, like The Prodigal Son, I lost interest in the Church. It seemed archaic and out of touch and the media (including Hollywood and the music industry) have done a good job of undermining religion. I call female singers like Madonna, Beyonce and Lady Ga Ga, 'Satan's little helpers'. These Baphomet Belles, crucifixes around their necks, dress like sluts and shriek, while pumping their hips and grabbing their crotches, spellbinding millions of pre-teens. I cannot save their sorry souls but a prescription should help with their crabs.

In the UK only about 4% of the population remain regular Churchgoers. You know the Anglican Church is lost when missionaries start coming to the UK, from Africa. How did the four great World religions get to be as popular and powerful as they are? Despite all the negative stories we hear, which are often nothing to do with religion but corrupt individuals within it, maybe, just maybe, they know something we do not. Is it possible Miracle Cures exist? There are examples. Every 'incurable' disease cured is, if you think about it, a miracle. I would like to introduce someone who knows a little about miracles. My daughter, Lauren.

The Last Rites

In 1990, Lauren was born, seven weeks premature, in a **British Military Hospital**, in Hong Kong. She weighed 3lb 4oz. The fact she was born at all was itself a miracle. A Naval surgeon in Hong Kong (I was based there at the time) had conducted a D&C (scraped the womb) of her mother, when 8 weeks pregnant. How he missed a 1" foetus we will never know. My wife knew she was pregnant (she had our son, Michael, previously) and two over-the-counter (OTC) pregnancy tests were positive. Unfortunately, the hospital's pregnancy test was negative, so that was that. They would not listen and went ahead with the procedure. My wife was devastated, believing she had lost her child. What relief we felt when her belly continued to swell. Although followed weeks of worry, wondering if the foetus had been damaged. A later complaint by us led to the hospital updating their tests.

Lauren was duly delivered, fingers and toes intact. Within days of her birth, she contracted double pneumonia. Her lungs became so stiff the incubator in the Special Care Baby Unit could not inflate them. She had to be hand-ventilated by nurses, round the clock. At one point her lungs burst, like balloons, with the pressure. One morning, around 4am, the hospital called us.

"Please come quickly! She will not last the hour".

In dread, we rushed to the hospital, arriving just before the final moments. Our daughter lay, grey and lifeless, her major organs failing. The Doctors had made every effort to save her, even injecting adrenaline directly into her heart. I looked at them. They shook their heads. The end was close. A kindly priest had rushed to administer the last rites. I was stunned. This could not be happening. Consumed with grief, I cried:

"God, please save her!"

The words came out as an unintelligible howl of anguish. Then something happened no-one has been able to explain. Within seconds, Lauren's failing heart rallied, then grew stronger. She survived.

"Watch me Catch a Crab!"

Four years later, I flew the children to America to visit the theme parks. Disneyland, SeaWorld, Universal Studios and so on. At one point in the holiday we drove up to Washington State to visit my wife's hermit-like father who lived in a small log cabin, on the edge of a lake. A charming man, he showed the children how to catch crabs by attaching chicken legs to a hook, then casting them into the lake, from the jetty. They loved it, as most children would. I was sat up at the house, watching, when Lauren called out:

"Daddy! Daddy! Watch me catch a crab!"

Lauren cast into the water and, to my horror, still holding the rod, followed the chicken into the lake. I raced down from the house as she disappeared under the surface and, eyes glued to the spot she went under, watched to see if she came up. She didn't. I dived in, desperately feeling around, water too murky to see anything. Dread enveloped me. So many children drown in these lakes. My searching became desperate. I came up for air then plunged down again. At this point, even if I did find her, would she still be alive? It felt like an eternity passed, as I frantically groped for her.

"I can't find her. I can't find her. Please, God. PLEASE God. Help me! HELP me!"

Then, suddenly, I felt a strand of hair, grabbed more, and then knew I had her. Thrusting as hard as I could, we surfaced. Watching Lauren's lungs empty of water, then breathe, was an indescribable relief. Later my son and I tried to make light of the incident by buying her a crab pendant with moving claws, to commemorate the occasion. It is perhaps fanciful of me to wonder if she still has it.

Supernatural Peace of Mind

I still pinch myself at what happened that night, in a quiet, countryside, English Abbey. For a decade I had suffered chronic anxiety, panic disorder and depression, trying all kinds of therapies, with little progress. Then, in one remarkable night, it was gone. The anxiety, panic, suicidal thinking, and depression. All of it. Replaced by an indescribable peace of mind and sense of wellbeing. How was this possible?

Like many people today, apart from Baptism and a Church wedding, my relationship with the Christian Church was non-existent. Feeling the strain of our daughter's struggle for life, I had started making tentative steps toward the Church. For the next 4 years, I was like a fish on a hook, slowly being reeled in. Why was it so difficult for me to embrace the Church? I needed to meet people who spoke normally and acted normally. People not driven by Messianic zeal to convert me.

Later, after re-marriage, I went from Church to Church, attending evangelical revivals, some of which were truly inspirational. Yet I couldn't bring myself to commit to what was on offer. Speaking in tongues, falling down, on cue, singing 'happy-clappy' tunes, raising hands high in the air and hugging strangers my instincts told me I should get away from as quickly as possible. My chest was too tight, voice too monotone and personality too introvert to play singalong.

One day my wife and I were invited to a 'Marriage Review' weekend run by CARE, a charity which supports family life. A series of workshops had been arranged to breathe life into stale and stuffy priests' ossified marriages. Our own marriage was in serious trouble, despite providing pre-marriage counselling to love-struck youngsters, with no clue what they were getting into. They were 'in love' and thought love was all that was needed for marital success. John Lennon was wrong when he wrote 'All You Need is Love'. Money is the number one cause of divorce.

The instructors for the course were refreshingly down-to-earth people. One in particular impressed me. I explained my chronic stress problems to him and how I could not understand why I wasn't able to bounce back. He related his own experience of anxiety. Born in a Japanese prisoner-of-war camp, his parents had been executed. He presented a simple choice:

"It is up to you. You can spend eight years with a psychiatrist and get nowhere or spend eight minutes with God and be transformed".

Hmm… This is what you call a 'no-brainer'. It was crunch time. Nothing ventured, nothing gained. After the workshop completed, I went to a room and this compassionate man led me through a brief, spoken ritual, with me basically saying…

"Father, I do not have the strength to do this alone, the burden is too heavy. From this point on I hand everything over to Jesus".

The experience was rather disappointing. There was no heavenly host of angels. No flashes of lightning. No transcendent experience with Jesus standing before me, holes in his hands. I did recall something highly unusual, though. My mind was screaming at me not to do it. I almost capitulated and walked out. Instead I did something I had never considered before. I told my mind to "Shut up!"

"Is that it?" I thought, and went to bed. The next morning, I was not the same person. I cannot recall a time, throughout my life, where my mind was ever at peace. It was always over-active, churning, out of control. Some have labelled this the 'Monkey Mind'. Buddha described the human mind as being filled with drunken monkeys, jumping around, screeching, chattering, carrying on endlessly. In Asia they say 'foreigners think too much'. They are right. Westerners have given primacy to the mind, to logic, reason and science. I saw my restless mind as a curse of intelligence. Now the worries, mental chatter and negative thinking which had been such an ever-present part of my life, were gone. Replaced by absolute peace of mind and an incredible feeling, as if floating on air.

I tried to rationalize what had happened. Handing your problems over to someone else will naturally lighten your burden. It is logical. Yet, this was something very different. A supernatural peace. What the Bible calls 'The Peace that Passeth all Understanding'. It cannot be explained. You have to experience it.

American Billy Graham was a charismatic, Christian evangelist and Spiritual adviser to several U.S. Presidents. Billy knew how to work a crowd. At large rallies, he would speak and encourage people to come forward to be converted. More than 3 million did so, over the years. After one particular religious revival, those who had come forward were asked later about their conversion experience. Most said their ecstatic state lasted about two months, before evaporating. Those, whose transformations were permanent, had immersed themselves in Christian life. They became selfless instead of selfish, helped others, read their Bible, joined the Church, prayed, and gave thanks to God for their salvation. They did not do as I did and ride the feeling, thinking it would last forever. Priests would tell me how blessed I was and to hang on to it. I did not understand what they meant. Once it was gone, I did. It is the same phenomenon I experienced in retreats. When you remain in a Church, Ashram, healing retreat, detox centre or gym, it is easy to stay on track. You have support from those around you, access to knowledge and the feeling of being part of one large family. However, once you leave, you become like a hot coal which jumps out of a roaring fire. Away from the heat, it quickly goes cold. You struggle to stay on the path and maintain changes. Enthusiasm and interest fade.

I am sure that incredible peace would have lasted longer, had I stayed within a supportive environment (this is why we provide follow-up support to those who attend our Retreats). Instead I could not overcome the difficulties I had with organized religion. I felt closer to 'God' sat under a tree than on a Church pew. The conflicts in my 'rebound' marriage had not resolved and my career in Information Technology came with 'Expect Burn-Out' in the Job Description. All these things and more chipped away at my supernatural peace, until it was gone, never to return. My 'miraculous' transformation had lasted nine months.

First Rule of Health

Whatever you are doing that is making you sick, STOP DOING IT!

A famous Indian Swami (holy man) listened to me, patiently, for over an hour, relating my tale of personal woe. Once off my chest, I waited expectantly for this wise man to deliver his sage advice. Drawn, perhaps, from the famous Bhagavad Gita, Upanishads or Vedas. The holy man spoke thus:

"Stop it".

I waited, breath suspended, for more wisdom to pour forth. The Swami turned away, the meeting clearly finished. Boy, was I disappointed. Today, I have come to realize what the Swami said to me was, in fact, the First Rule of Health. Do any of the following sound familiar?

"I know junk food is making me ill but I love it".

"I need my cigarette/chocolate/beer/coffee/computer games, to help me relax".

"What they show on TV makes me so angry/worried/sad"

"I know I should exercise more but..."

"I really should be more positive but..."

You get the idea. Most of us know already what is making us sick. The answer, as the holy man pointed out, is to:

STOP eating garbage, drinking and staying up too late.

STOP watching TV if it disturbs you.

STOP being a couch-potato, negative, or arguing with each other.

STOP whatever you are doing that is making you sick!

Only when you STOP building disease can you START to build health.

Second Rule of Health

Whatever you are doing that is making you sick, DO THE OPPOSITE!

Ayurveda has two simple laws.

1. Law of Similars

2. Law of Opposites.

How do they work? Very simply:

Similars

If I am fat and eat fattening food, I will become fatter.

If I am slim and eat slimming foods, I will become slimmer.

If I am cold and eat cooling foods, I will feel colder.

If I am hot and eat heating foods, I will become hotter.

If I am dry and eat drying foods, I will become drier.

If I am wet and eat watery foods, I will become wetter.

Opposites

If I am fat and eat reducing foods, I will become slimmer.

If I am slim and eat fattening foods, I will become fatter.

If I am cold and eat heating foods, I will feel warmer.

If I am hot and eat cooling foods, I will become cooler.

If I am dry and eat watery foods, I will become wetter.

If I am wet and eat drying foods, I will become drier.

As you can see, when trying to restore health, it is not just a matter of stopping what you are doing but doing the opposite. This applies equally to our emotions and thought processes. Think about how these laws might apply in your own life.

Cure Yourself

Numerous health books tell you how to cure this or that disease. They generally describe the condition, then provide the cure. This is not that type of book because authentic natural healing is not symptom-based. It is vitalist and holistic. Not focused on symptoms (disease labels) but underlying cause. My intention is to first give you a proper understanding of why you need to rely on yourself, then provide a handful of methods which have been reported as healing almost all conditions.

There are thousands of anecdotes, online and in print, from those cured of chronic disorders. Take cancer. There are at least 350 natural cancer cures and hundreds of herbs and foods with proven anti-cancer activity. Renee Caisse and Harold Hoxsey are famous (to those who have researched them) for curing many thousands of cancer patients, using herbal formulas, over several decades. Renee Caisse was seeing 300-500 patients per week for years. Harry Hoxsey had 17 thriving clinics and the support of patients, congressmen and even some Doctors.

Dr Richard Schulze also cured thousands of the most severe cases before he was shut down. I could list a dozen other practitioners who also had good results with cancer over the years, who were persecuted and shut down. Actress Susan Somers says she was cured of breast cancer with 'Iscador' (Mistletoe). Mistletoe has been known to cure cancer, for 100 years, yet few people know. Likewise, Laetrile (B17). Shark Cartilage is documented as stopping cancer from spreading (angiogenesis). Raw garlic, the same. **Dr Tullio Simoncini**, an Italian oncologist (Cancer doctor), says fungi are at the heart of every tumour. He has numerous testimonies, from those who assert they were cured of cancer, using $3 worth of baking soda (kills fungi). Interestingly, baking soda is recorded as a cancer cure in 1000 year old Ayurvedic texts. The average cancer treatment costs $350,000 per patient and baking soda only $3. That is a mighty powerful incentive to dismiss and suppress Dr Simoncini's protocol. If such a 'miracle' cancer cure were to be accepted and recognized, the $multi-billion cancer industry might collapse.

'This treatment was developed in Italy by an oncologist and uses baking soda or sodium bicarbonate. This treatment is primarily used for cancer of the digestive tract, including cancers of the throat, colon, intestines, rectal area, and other cancers in between. Cancers outside of the digestive tract generally need a health practitioner to inject the baking soda solution.'

https://www.cancertutor.com/simoncini/

One question I am sometimes asked is, "Which is better for health. Fruits or vegetables?" Naturopath Dr Robert Morse is a brilliant naturopath who regards vegetables as builders, repairers and regenerators, suited for muscle and skeletal tissue. Whereas fruits are brain and nerve foods as well as cleansers of tissue. Fruits have the highest electrical energy of all the foods. The more energetic the foods you eat, the more vibrant and healthy you become. If I want to give my body a spring clean, I consume fruits or their juices. If I am trying to heal or regenerate tissue, it's vegetable juices. Nuts and seeds are structural foods, strengthening the body as a whole.

The Essiac and Hoxsey herbal formulas. The Budwig Diet, Baking Soda, Gerson Therapy, the naturopathic methods of Richard Schulze and the Ornish Heart program. All super contenders for healing. Since it is impossible to cover all possibilities, I will limit myself to just four.

Let's start with the basics. Recovering your health is like renovating a home. If you feel like a dilapidated building, with crumbling foundations, you are going to need some restoration. Restoration of any structure requires planning. Consider some of the elements you need:

1. Good architectural design (Your healing program).

2. Materials (Supplements, herbs, supportive therapies).

3. A Project Manager, to keep reconstruction on schedule; come rain or shine. (Health Coach/friend/family member).

4. Prepare the ground (Cleanse and detoxify).

5. Put in strong foundations (Flood the body with nutrients).

6. Build the walls, put on the roof and install plumbing, electrics and windows (The 5 Layers of Healing).

7. Keep your home in good order. (Healthy lifestyle, resolve minor problems before they become serious disorders).

For those who are highly stressed, easily discouraged or seeking instant fixes, this may already seem like hard work. It is not. The only difficulty is having the confidence and motivation to get on with it.

What Are The Methods?

1. **Water Cure**. As simple and affordable as you can get.

2. **Reversing Diabetes**. Equally simple. On our 'Reverse Diabetes' retreats, I have observed conditions like Type II Diabetes and pre-diabetes (hypoglycaemia, hyperglycemia and metabolic disorder) reverse within 7 days and be 100% resolved, within 21, just by a change in nutrition. Dr Gabriel Cousens at the Tree of Life Centre, Arizona, has been curing Type II Diabetes with his raw food program, for 30 years.

3. **Auto-Urine Therapy**. This will surprise you.

4. **'Incurables' Program**. The core of the healing protocol I used to cure myself and which can be applied to just about every chronic and degenerative disorder that exists.

The Incurables program is based on a protocol by Dr John Christopher and his student, Dr Richard Schulze (a Naturopath and Master Herbalist in the U.S.) who used it to "save the lives of thousands of extremely sick people". Both practitioners became well known (and persecuted) for curing those, conventional and alternative medicine could not help. The 'Incurables' is a 30-day program, incorporating many classical naturopathic steps. You may not need all 30 days or you may need longer. It depends how well you apply the program and the nature of your disorder. For a more in-depth look, I highly recommend Richard's books.

All the above can be undertaken at home. The latter has more steps. However, each step is easy to understand and apply. If you recall, at the beginning of the book, Dan's Rheumatoid Arthritis symptoms were gone in 14 days. If you are not seeing results like this, you may be doing something wrong. Oftentimes you may be following the program correctly but are not aggressive enough with your approach. A well-designed holistic Detox/Cleanse is at the core of all Natural healing systems, including the 'Incurables' program. Remember Dr Richard Schulze's statement 80% of disorders will resolve by properly cleaning the bowel? In my experience, for most conditions, 10 days is the minimum time needed to start seeing results with chronic disorders. It is also the minimum time recommended to kill off parasites and fungi. Standard anti-Candida protocols will kill fungi (also known as thrush or yeast infection) but are often complicated and can take 3 months or more to work. Because of this they often fail. It is quicker and more effective to fast (read Angela's story). A parasite cleanse also needs a little thought. People can be host to a variety of different parasites including flukes, amoeba, giardia, pinworms and tapeworms. You can find parasite-cleanse preparations, online. It takes about 6 weeks to remove parasites and their eggs from the body.

Your healing outcome is very much dependent on you. If you are prepared to give it 100% you will be giving the best possible support to your body's innate healing efforts. A one month commitment is nothing compared to years of continued illness and far less dangerous than a stay in hospital. No matter how quick or convenient.

Using the house fire analogy again, how would you feel if your house was on fire and someone turned up with a squirt-gun? Wouldn't you want as may fire hoses as possible? Wouldn't you wish them to keep hosing the smouldering members until you were sure the fire was out and couldn't re-ignite? The 'Incurables' program operates on the same principle. Attacking the disease process in a sustained way and keeping attacking until your disorder is resolved. It is designed to produce rapid results. You can achieve similar outcomes, over a longer period, with a raw, organic, vegan diet. However, in my opinion, the shorter the timescale, the less chance of self-sabotage. As Dan from Canada said:

"There are quick, medium and slow ways to restore health. All have their advantages and disadvantages. It seemed preferable, at least to me, if I am going to forego all my treats, in order for my health to be restored, I would rather get it over with quickly."

The 'Incurables' protocol requires you to juice-fast for the whole 30 days, if possible. You can choose to do this alone. However, I would strongly suggest you find a professional, with experience of fasting, to monitor you.

Fasting or Starving?

Confusion exists; usually among those who have never tried it, that fasting and starvation are one and the same. They are not. Fasting is defined as follows:

'The voluntary denial of food to a system which is diseased, and which, because of disease, does not require nourishment until rested, cleansed, and the digestive 'fire' restored. Then, and not till then, is food supplied; then, and not till then, does starvation begin.'

In short, fast until you are cured. Once cured, eat again.

What is the 'digestive fire'? This is another name for appetite. In Ayurveda, the concept of 'fire' and digestion is crucial. Try an experiment. Wait until hungry, then consume an ice-cream or chilled drink. Your hunger will go. You have extinguished your digestive 'fire'. If you then eat, food becomes harder to break down because fats have solidified, digestion will take longer and more energy is consumed. Frozen products and iced drinks are unnatural. If your appetite is weak, you need to be stoking the 'fire' with warming herbs and spices. Not extinguishing it.

When we are unwell, our bodies tell us to stop eating. We lose our appetite. However, due to addiction, habit or ignorance, we continue to eat. We even force our sick children to eat when they do not wish to. Telling them it is to 'keep your strength up'. When you eat without hunger, food becomes toxic to the body, fermenting and putrefying in the intestinal tract, producing toxins which are then taken up by the blood and deposited in other areas of the body such as the joints. Stress is placed upon our organs which not only have to cope with our disorders but an additional toxic burden.

When you drink freshly squeezed, organic fruit or vegetable juices during a fast, you are not starving. You are still delivering nutrients to your cells. Juicing simply removes the fibre. To reduce weight loss, juice combinations can be designed to be higher in calories. The classic 'Master Cleanse' includes organic maple syrup, which provides around 400 calories per day. You can increase or decrease the amount of maple syrup, as desired, and therefore the calories. I do not recommend commercial maple syrup since it is difficult to find truly organic versions. Instead I substitute freshly squeezed Sugar-Cane juice, which is available locally. In some programs I would not use sugars at all, except Stevia, such as an Anti-Candida fast.

What caused us to be sick in the first place? The main source of symptoms of disease is impure blood. Impure blood is caused by impaired digestion. Poor eating habits, incorrect food choices and eating more than is needed for repair and growth of tissue cells. In all three instances, the resolution is to stop eating, clean up the system, reset the digestion and correct eating habits. Historically this has been done by fasting, sometimes assisted by additional treatments, such as bodywork and steam baths. The ancient Roman Baths and Baden Baden, in Germany, have wonderful mineral baths.

How Long and How Often Should You Fast?

Jesus fasted for 40 days and 40 nights. Pythagoras fasted his students for 21 days, to make their minds sharper. Some fast until the tongue is clean. Others until their disease has resolved. I would look at the condition, capacity and willingness of the individual. Some are happy to continue until healed. Some take a break then repeat the fast later. 15 years ago, the recommendation was, we should fast at regular intervals, such as the changing of the seasons. I used to recommend this myself. However, since we are being poisoned by chemicals, on a daily basis, that advice is somewhat inadequate. We need to make the elimination of toxins a daily routine. Reducing the amount of toxins coming in, as well as adopting a detoxifying diet. We can juice organic vegetables and/or fruits or drink 'detox' tea. Detoxification from heavy metals, fluoride, chemicals, radiation and vaccines, is a specialist subject that needs to be addressed separately.

Which Juices?

Over many 100's of years, natural healing practitioners have learned which fruit and vegetable combinations are best suited to particular conditions. If you watch TV or follow celebrity juicing experts, you will be dazzled by their creativity and the juice combinations they present. They do a great job but, like circus acts, tend to over-egg the pudding. They want to stay relevant, make a name for themselves and keep people interested. Some of their creations I would not consider appropriate for healing. Our 7-day and 21-day 'Super Juice!' retreats include fruit and vegetable shakes, using a wonderful array of organic fruits and vegetables, grown locally and picked fresh.

Since fruits are better than vegetables for cleansing, we tend to use fruit juices for detoxing, sometimes selecting particular fruits for specific conditions. 'The Master Cleanse' using the cleansing power of citrus, is classic for conditions like arthritis. We fall back on water-only fasts if juices do not appear to be working, guests specifically request them or individuals are sensitive to juices. Spiritual practitioners use water-only fasts for purification and to help reach enlightened states. Dry fasts are little known but can be added to protocols to accelerate a cleanse. Like wringing out a sponge.

Many and varied are the possibilities. Have Candida? Try a Colloidal Silver fast, an Apple Cider Vinegar fast or a young coconut water fast. We select only what is in season. There are juices specific to Arthritis and juices specific to cancer. When someone comes for a Yoga Holiday, or is convalescing, we can provide tasty fruit shakes. However, for healing-related programs, liquids are preferred to solids. This accords with the ancients view that, in order to recover one's health, you must stop eating altogether. You can still enjoy the shakes but ONLY after your healing program is finished. It is important, when starting any juice or water fast, to start gently and finish gently. For pre-fast, eat soft fruits and steamed vegetables. This takes the burden off digestion and prepares the body for the start of the fast. Stop eating anything that is difficult for the digestive system to break down, such as meat, at least 24 hours before you commence your program. It is also necessary to break the fast, correctly. After the fast, eat only soft fruits and steamed vegetables, like pumpkin, for two days. After not eating for a week or more, they taste divine!

What is Ketosis?

You may have heard of Ketosis or a Ketogenic Diet. It is becoming very popular but is basically the Atkins Diet revisited. Instead of burning carbs for energy, the body switches over to burning fats (ketone bodies). A low carbohydrate, high fat (LCHF) program is an example of a ketogenic diet.

Ketosis occurs when the body does not have enough glucose for energy. Instead, stored fats are broken down and converted to glucose, while toxins and waste matter are released from fat stores and excreted. Dr Nicholas Gonzalez, known for treating cancers and chronic disease, using individualized nutrition, fasting, supplements and digestive enzymes, became very familiar with Dr Atkins and his successes. He reports the Atkins Diet was not just a weight-loss diet. It cured a number of disorders. However, it was not very successful with Cancer. Beware the internet echo-chamber. It could be the Ketogenic Diet is not, as some claim, the best diet for Cancer. If anyone has examples of it healing cancer, please let me know.

Frank Tippett

Frank Tippett was diagnosed with Multiple Sclerosis (MS) in April 2000. MRIs showed the myelin sheath missing and plaque on the brain. Frank suffered numbness, tingling, pain, slurred speech, a loss of control of his right arm, walking and balance problems, his bodily functions slowed down and he was constantly tired.

The doctor put Frank on Avonex, which helped for three days out of the week. This became longer, once Frank started a Water Cure. He also took cold-pressed flax seed oil, B Complex, lecithin, a one-a-day vitamin, and potassium. Two and a half months after Frank started the Water Cure his numbness and tingling were gone. In the following months his walking and balance improved and bodily functions returned to normal. In December 2001 he came off the Avonex. All the tests for MS showed he was in excellent health. As an added bonus, Frank had an enlarged prostate for seven years. His family doctor checked it during his last visit and reported it as normal. Frank feels to deal with the effects of MS you need a positive attitude, an open mind and a willingness to try other treatments, like the Water Cure.

"I haven't felt this good in twenty years", says Frank. "Thanks to Dr. Batmanghelidj".

Water Cures

For legal reasons, I will remind you of the disclaimer at the beginning of the book. If you have any serious medical condition, especially involving your kidneys, you should not attempt a water cure without first consulting your Doctor. In fact, sharing this information with your Doctor is highly recommended. Anyone attempting cures mentioned in this book, do so of their own volition. I present them for educational purposes only.

In his bestselling book Your Body's Many Cries for Water, Dr. F. Batmanghelidj (a conventional medical Doctor) explains the cause of many of today's disorders, including pain and Cancer, is chronic dehydration. In his books he provides scholarly examples of conditions cured by increasing fluid intake. One health writer had this to say about Dr. Batmanghelidj's follow-up book 'Water Cures. Drugs Kill'

"...after a wake-up call to America and Britain, Dr. B outlines several disease states (warning symptoms) which progress to actual damage. He elaborates multiple and varied case histories which confirm dehydration as the cause of symptoms. His examples are so varied almost anyone could find, within the pages of his books, information directly relevant to his/her personal situation."

The message we receive from Dr. Batmanghelidj is you are not only what you eat but also what you drink. (I might add 'you are what you are able to assimilate.') Since water is assimilated easily and rapidly, it is the perfect treatment. Not only that, it costs pennies. How many of us drink water? You will be surprised at the number who don't. When I ask why, the answer given is usually they do not like the taste. I can sympathize. Some municipal and bottled waters do not taste clean. There is no glacier water in my area, nor running, dancing, gurgling, mineral springs. If there is, a drinks giant has stuck a bottling plant on it. Finding pure water today is almost impossible.

Let's touch on how much of our bodies are made up of water.

Muscles 75%.

Blood 82%.

Lungs 90%.

Brain 76%.

Bones 25%.

Our lymphatic system, which transports waste from our bodies, cannot do so without adequate water. Many of us are dehydrated, do not know it and do not realize many disorders are caused by a lack of sufficient water. Why are detox and cleansing programs effective in resolving these disorders? Because they flood our tissues with fluid. Even using juices, we are hydrating our tissues. Remember the sponge analogy? Put a dirty sponge in a bucket of water overnight and in the morning the sponge will be clean, the dirt sitting on the bottom of the bucket. The water has lifted the dirt from the sponge. What would happen if there were insufficient water in the bucket? The sponge would stay dirty. Likewise, our bodies. By not drinking sufficient water, we cause 'dirt' to accumulate, restricting the lymphatic (drainage) system's ability to mobilize waste and transport it to our organs of elimination. Hippocrates tells us that anything in excess is bad for us. Conversely, anything which is deficient is also bad for us. Dehydration causes deficiency diseases. Water and juice fasts flood the tissues with water, reversing deficiency, resolving the root cause of our disorders.

How Long Should We Drink Extra Fluid?

If too little water makes me sick, won't too much? Yes. Which is why people only undertake these protocols until the body is clean and the disease condition resolved.

I Can't Drink That Much Water!

Some people have difficulty when they try to increase their fluid intake. I sympathize. Being a dry 'Air' type, I find it difficult to take in large amounts of fluids, so build up slowly or drink water throughout the day.

Water Cure 1

Drink 1.5 litres of clean water, on an empty stomach, on rising, then do not eat or drink for the following hour. Do this 3x daily, for 1 week, for Arthritis and Rheumatism, then 2x daily until you are healed. For all other disorders, 2x daily is recommended.

Water Cure 2

This cure comes from Dr Batmanghelidj who has conducted a great deal of research to back up his claims. He says to drink 8 glasses of water per day, with ½ teaspoon of sea salt. Around 1/8th level teaspoon of sea salt to each 8oz glass. Use uniodized sea salt or Celtic sea salt.

Why Don't We Know About Water Cures?

Water cannot be patented. It seems too simple. Health professionals can hardly charge for them.

It Isn't Working!

Years of observation demonstrate that some conditions are stubborn. Often due to a failure of the individual to disclose important information, or failing to follow ALL the steps necessary to recover health. Picking and choosing the steps they like, while ignoring the steps they don't. If the Water Cure is not working for you, I would give it a helping hand. Look to improve those other aspects of your health you may be neglecting. Diet, exercise and stress reduction. The same applies to oxygen therapies.

If you are struggling, don't give up, telling yourself 'I'll never be cured!" Look at what you may be doing wrong or a step you might have missed. If it still isn't working, there are always alternatives. Call the cavalry and seek support. Find a Naturopath or Ayurvedic Doctor or call me and I can see what you are doing. Never lose hope!

A Most Unexpected Cure

I must have a mischievous streak. With all the possibilities to choose from, I pick the one most likely to induce you to toss this book in the trash.

Have you ever tasted or drank your own urine? "Yuck!" I hear you say. Why would anyone do that? It is a waste product, surely? Dirty, smelly and dangerous.

'Urine therapy' is an ancient healing practice which has fallen out of favour in the last 150 years. Well, almost. You will be surprised to learn urine is still used, medicinally, today. Urine is an ingredient in a number of products, such as face cream. Its origin disguised, using innocent-sounding labels. In Ayurveda they call urine, 'Shivambu Shastra' which means "Water of Shiva", a very auspicious name. There is even an annual World Conference on Urine Therapy, attended by scholars.

Why would I even consider drinking my own urine? Well, desperation, mostly, and curiosity. Frustrated with my failure to recover, I came across a book with a remarkable story to tell. '**Your Own Perfect Medicine**' by Martha Christy.

The following, is from Biomedx:

Ms. Christy was sick. Very sick. For a very long time. Pelvic inflammatory disease, ulcerative colitis, Chron's disease, chronic fatigue syndrome, Hashimoto's disease, mononucleosis. She had severe kidney infections, two miscarriages, chronic cystitis, severe candida, endometriosis, adrenal insufficiency, serious chronic ear and sinus infections, food and chemical allergies. That wasn't the half of it. Martha had every conceivable medical test, her share of surgery, and drugs - plenty of them. Then she tried all forms of alternative therapy. Homeopathy, herbs, mega-vitamins and liv-cell treatments in Mexico. After traditional medicine failed to work, she and her husband spent over $100,000 trying to get her well with alternative approaches. Nothing worked.

And then one day, her husband brought home a little book that told of how individuals had been cured of even the worst diseases with a seemingly strange and little-known natural therapy. Soon afterwards, she began the therapy herself. From the first day she began, she received almost instantaneous relief from her incurable constipation and fluid retention. Within a week, her severe abdominal and pelvic pain was gone.

The chronic cystitis and yeast infections (internal and external) soon disappeared and her food allergies, exhaustion, and digestive problems all began to heal.

After a few more months, her colds, flu, sore throats and on again, off again viral symptoms disappeared. Her hair which had fallen out by the handfuls after her fifth surgery became thick and lustrous. Her weight normalized, and her energy and strength came back. After nearly 30 years of non-stop illness, Martha Christy was whole again.

The incredible 'Miracle Cure' Martha discovered? Her own urine.

Let's get the main objection out of the way. The smell. If your diet is healthy, your output does not smell like a public toilet in an Irish bar. Your urine has virtually no scent, or taste, and runs almost clear. "A hint of summer meadows" I used to joke with friends. Urine is not what we think it is. In her book, Martha Christy explains:

Urine is not, as many believe, the excess water from food and liquids that goes through the intestines and is ejected from the body as "waste". It is much different and much more. When you eat, the food you ingest is eventually broken down in the stomach and intestines into extremely small molecules. These molecules are absorbed into tiny tubules in the intestinal wall and then pass through these tubes into the blood stream.

The blood circulates throughout your body carrying these food molecules and other nutrients, along with critical immune defense and regulating elements such as red and white blood cells, antibodies, plasma, microscopic proteins, hormones, enzymes, etc., which are all manufactured at different locations in the body.

As the blood circulates, it passes through the liver where toxins are removed and later excreted from the body in the form of solid waste. Eventually, this now purified "cleaned" blood makes its way to the kidneys. When blood enters the kidneys it is filtered through an immensely complex and intricate system of minute tubules called nephron through which the blood is literally "squeezed" at high pressure. This filtering process removes excess amounts of water, salts and other elements in the blood your body does not need at the time.

These excess elements are collected within the kidney in the form of a purified, sterile, watery solution called urine. Many of the constituents of this filtered watery solution, or urine, are then reabsorbed by the nephron and delivered back into the bloodstream. The remainder of the urine passes out of the kidneys into the bladder and is then excreted from the body.

The function of the kidneys is to keep the various elements in your blood balanced. When your body doesn't need something at a particular time, it is excreted - not because it is toxic or poisonous or bad for the body, but simply because the body does not need that particular element at the time.

Medical researchers have discovered many of the elements of the blood, found in urine, have enormous medicinal value, and when reintroduced to the body, boost the body's immune defences and stimulate healing in a way nothing else does.

You may not realize it but you are probably already absorbing someone else's urine into your cells. 'Pergonal' is a fertility drug made from human urine. 'Urokinase', a urine ingredient, is sold as a blood clot dissolver for unblocking coronary arteries. Urea, medically proven to be one of the best moisturizers in the world, is packaged in expensive creams and lotions and is approved by the FDA. Take the M out of 'Murine' eye drops and what do you have? Claims have been made urine can cure over 175 different diseases. Martha went on to investigate the use of urine therapy around the world and reports its use is far more prevalent than most of us realize. Many people have come to her disclosing their own healing experiences, particularly with allergies. Beginning to understand urine is safe, a potential 'cure-all' and life-saver?

How to take it? The following is a suggested routine.

Day 1. 1-5 drops (of morning, mid-stream urine)

Day 2. 5-10 drops in the morning.

Day 3. 5-10 drops in the morning and evening.

Gradually increase the amount as needed, to obtain results for your condition. Work up to drinking an ounce or two at a time. Oh yes. Expect to get seriously ribbed by friends and family. Treat it with a little humour. We are far too serious. When I was experimenting with friends, we had a great time making jokes about our newly discovered auto-urine therapy. Let me know how the 'amber nectar' works for you.

"Bottoms up!"

Carlos Cervantes

In July 2008 Carlos Cervantes was diagnosed with Type II Diabetes. His fasting blood sugar was over 500 (28 mmol/l) and he was experiencing thirst, constant tiredness and felt like he was in a kind of semi-comatose state. Metformin caused him to gain 30lbs, so he switched to Glipizide, where he gained another 5lbs. In 2010, after 6 months of a diabetic-driven ear infection, Carlos was put on insulin. In December Carlos developed his first diabetic foot ulcer, then a second in June 2011, so serious he faced amputation. There were problems with his kidneys, liver and eyesight, and painful neuropathy in his feet. In Feb 2011 Carlos had a heart attack. 3 months later his insulin dose was increased by his Doctor. By this point, Carlos accepted he was going to die. A higher power, apparently, had other ideas and 3 hours later, Carlos was drawn to a 2-minute news item which completely turned him around. It was about a Newcastle University Study, where a group of Type 2 Diabetics, led by Professor Roy Taylor, had completely reversed their diabetes within 8 weeks. How had this 'miracle' been achieved? A reduced-calorie diet and exercise.

Carlos decided to try the Newcastle Study diet but instead of 800 calories per day, opted for 600, for 64 days. Carlos has said, during interviews, he found it pretty tough. Doctors know 90% or more of people who attempt such diets, give up. But Carlos, to his credit, was very determined. Adopting soups, salads, lots of water and a little gentle walking. On the 18th of July 2011, the day after starting the program, Carlos stopped his insulin completely. Within 11 days his blood sugar readings were normal. Today, Carlos is healthy. His blood sugar levels range from 67-73 (approx. 3.7 mmol/l) and all his diabetic symptoms have disappeared. He weighs 174 lbs. Dramatically down from a high of 305lbs.

Reversing Diabetes

Every 30 seconds a lower limb is amputated as a consequence of diabetes. Yet, ample evidence has existed, for at least 40 years, Type 2 Diabetes can be reversed, with nutrition alone. Mainstream support for this comes from the 2011 Newcastle Study (a few decades behind but never mind). Type 2 Diabetes is one of the easier disorders to resolve because Type 2 Diabetes is a LIFESTYLE disease. Caused by what we are putting in our mouths.

At Antarana, believe juice-fasting to be superior and easier to stick to than eating raw food, since, and this may surprise you, there is less hunger during fasting. Alongside cleansing, bodywork, herbs, hydrotherapy and Ayurvedic methods like 'Shirodhara', fasting blood sugar normalizes within 1-4 days, excess fat is cleared from the liver and pancreatic function markedly improved or fully restored, within 21 days. Approximately 60% of non-insulin-dependent Type II Diabetics reverse their diabetes within 3 weeks, with the remainder doing so in subsequent weeks. Insulin-dependent Type II diabetes also see initial success (approx. 25%) coming off all insulin and other medications. Do diabetics need to attend a Retreat? No. But they may wish to. The fact is, without support, 9 out of 10 people will not stick to a healing program. If you have ever made a New Year Resolution, you will understand why. When facing a global pandemic of diabetes, there is an obvious need for 'Reverse Diabetes' Retreats, like ours.

Prediabetes

Hypoglycaemia, Hyperglycaemia and Metabolic Disorder (Syndrome X) are, together, known as prediabetes. Hypoglycaemia is a condition resulting from low blood sugar. Symptoms of hypoglycaemia can include food cravings, weakness, depression, insomnia and more. Many people treat hypoglycemia with sweets, biscuits, potato chips, chocolate, etc... to raise their sugar level quickly. This works - but only for a short period. When you take in food, high in carbohydrates or sugar, your body senses a sharp increase in blood sugar level and the pancreas produces insulin in response. Your sugar level plummets. You feel weak or shaky, so crave sugar again. Repeat this cycle continuously and your pancreas becomes worn-out and you are insulin-dependent, with full-blown diabetes. Yo-yoing like this is harmful and unnecessary.

Cure rate for prediabetes? 100% within 14 days.

The 30-Day Program

To recap. You are going to:

- Commit 100% to the program

- Stop whatever you are doing that is making you sick and reverse it. (Law of Similars & Opposites)

- Ensure your channels of elimination are open.

- Clear physical, emotional, psychological, energetic and spiritual blockages - The 5 Layers of Healing.

- Move your blood and lymph

- Balance your PH

- Provide proper cellular respiration (ensure enough oxygen is getting to your cells)

- Flood your body with nutrients

If this seems a little daunting, do not worry. Yes, it is easier to attend a retreat, where it is all set up for you but bear in mind this is a comprehensive (w)holistic program, based on not knowing the root cause of your disorder(s). If you have already identified the underlying cause of your condition, the full program may not be necessary. You may be healed just with bowel cleansing or a more targeted approach. Stick with it because by the time you are finished, you are going to feel transformed. Feeling better is not a hardship!

Assuming you have already taken Steps 1&2...

Step 3. Ensure your channels of elimination (bowels, lungs, liver, kidneys and skin) are open. The bowels need to be moving and emptied. This can be done with laxative teas like Senna; Castor Oil, Triphala (an herb), salt water flushes (using uniodized sea salt) or enemas. Enema kits can be bought in most pharmacies or health stores. Dr Richard Schulze has an online herbal store at www.herbdoc.com selling two intestinal formulas. The first is to get the bowels moving. If your bowels are moving okay (many people are constipated) you do not need it. The second formula assists in cleansing and restoring the colon and is a must.

Breathing exercises will strengthen and expand the lungs, get you breathing properly and bring in more oxygen, while expelling carbonic acid and other harmful wastes, stagnating at the bottom of your lungs. Flushes, for liver, gall bladder and kidneys, will eliminate toxins from those organs. Dry and wet skin-brushing clears blocked pores and gets your circulation and lymph moving.

Step 4. Address The 5 Layers. How to do this has been covered previously chapters. Please review EFT+NLP and 'Breaking The Chains'. Both of these techniques are easy to learn and apply at home.

Step 5. Is achieved with massage, contrast bathing and exercise.

Step 6. Vegetable juices will alkalize your tissues and expel acid wastes.

Step 7. Green juices with chlorophyll, breathing exercises, 3% Hydrogen Peroxide drops, are believed to not only oxidize pathogens (our body produces hydrogen peroxide to kill cancer cells) but will bring more oxygen to the cells. Ed McCabe's book 'Flood Your Body with Oxygen' has some great information.

Step 8. It is very hard to consume sufficient vegetable matter, in its raw state, to obtain needed amounts of nutrients. Munching through a plate of leafy greens is hard work. If you have digestive issues, you may not have enough digestive 'fire' to break down raw vegetables. Juicing them allows nutrients to be absorbed rapidly.

The following is an example Daily Schedule I use during a Detox/Healing Fast. There are many variations of juices and herbs, tailored for different conditions but those listed should do the job. Explanations for each step are given.

Watching the Scales

A word about weight loss. Some guests become obsessed by the scales, worrying they are not shedding weight they are desperate to lose. Understand that, at the beginning of any fast, while you may not see fat loss externally, accumulated fat internally (e.g. fatty liver) is being broken down and consumed. Rates of weight loss are different for each of us. We are not all the same. On average, people lose around 1/2 a kilo per day. If you are more active, it tends to be more. If you are sedentary, we much prefer you to not worry. Forget the scales and concentrate instead on becoming healthy.

TIME	DAILY SCHEDULE
0600	On rising, greet the day positively. Open arms wide and say "I FEEEEEEEL GREEEAAATTTT!!!"
0605	Dry Skin Brushing + beat yourself up! + Hot & Cold Shower (1 min Hot, 1 min Cold. 7x)
0630	Bitter Gourd, Cucumber, Tomato Juice OR Lemon Soda + Herbal Tincture
0700	Morning walk + deep breathing. Or swim + Pranayama in fresh morning air + stretching/Yoga
0800	'Mae West' retention enema
0900	8oz Nutrient Drink (Carrot, Apple, Garlic (2 cloves), Celery & Parsley) + Bentonite Shake
0905	Sun and wind-bathing + Sesame Oil
1000	Herbal Steam Sauna (10-30mins) followed by Ice water dip or shower. Skin brush + vigorous rub with towel. Potassium Broth
1030	Sesame Oil Massage + Deep Reflexology + Hot Herbal Bolus
1100	Detox Drink
1230	Hydrotherapy. Hot + Cold spinal hosing OR spinal immersion in cold water
1500	8oz Detox Drink + Tincture+ Bentonite Shake
1600	Sun + wind-bathing. Sesame Oil + drink water
1700	Potassium Broth + 30 minute walk, swim or Yoga. Breathe hard and encourage sweating.
1945	8oz Nutrient Drink (Carrot, Apple, Beetroot, Garlic (2 cloves), Celery & Parsley) + Bentonite Shake
2000	Relax

*Times are flexible. Adjust them to suit your needs:

Start the Day in the Right Way

Waking up grumpy? Never mind. Go to your bedroom window, throw open the curtains and shout out loudly "I FEEEEEEEL GREEEAAATTTT!!!" Fake it until you make it. Do it every morning. Some days you just can't do it. That's ok. Shut down, chill out. Tell yourself, "It's only a passing cloud".

Juicing

The simplest and most famous juice for detoxing comes from 'The Master Cleanse'. You only need organic lemons, some chilli powder and a natural sweetener. For reversing disease you want to be drinking one 8oz glass per hour. Use the juice of one lemon, in 8oz clean water, a pinch of chilli powder and Organic Maple Syrup or Sugar Cane Juice (to taste). That's it! When I detox, I drink a 16oz glass every 2 hours and take a carry-out with me if I am away from home.

A morning Lemon Soda is a great way to start the day, whether you are sick or not. Take the juice of 1 lemon and a ¼ tsp of baking soda in an 8oz glass of water and drink. Adding a pinch of chilli powder will dilate your arteries and assist in delivering the cleansing and healing factors around your body. Drinking these drinks hot (not scalding) is also highly beneficial. Cold or ice drinks shock the digestive system, put out your digestive fire and thicken fats. The opposite effect you are aiming for. We want fats and fluids to flow to our tissues smoothly, in the same way warm oil does in a car.

It is also important to drink water in between the juices. Keep those cells fully hydrated! What about juices specific to your condition? Please see the list of juices and conditions they address, at the end of this chapter.

Dry Skin Brushing

Brush your skin before you bath or shower. This stimulates the neuro-muscular system (invigorates you), improves blood circulation and stagnation in the lymphatic system and sloughs off dead skin. Use a loofah or firm (not too stiff) brush. Brush toward the heart. If you forget to brush when your skin is dry, use a wet brush in the shower or bath.

Beat Yourself Up!

Using the knuckles of a clenched fist, 'tap-tap-tap' all over your body. The idea is you are dislodging 'dirt' and blockages, as well as stimulating your circulation. Ask your partner to 'beat you up', or do the program together and beat each other up! It is a great way to bond. No bruising, please!

Herbal Steam Sauna

Herbal steam saunas enhance detoxification. At Antarana, we typically use 10 different herbs and sometimes add ozone. However, neither are strictly necessary, just as long as you are sweating. Different Constitutional Types benefit from different lengths of time in the sauna. Slim 'Air' types stay a maximum of 15 minutes. Hardy 'Fire' types, also 15 minutes (they get too heated). Heavy 'Earth' and 'Water' types can stay up to 30 minutes. When you exit, douse yourself or have a dip in cold water, to close the pores. Scandinavians have used Saunas, for detoxification, for centuries.

   Note: We do not use, nor recommend, FAR Infra-Red Saunas. Almost all FAR models have been found to emit unacceptable levels of radiation.

Breathing (Pranayama)

Many different breathing exercises exist, for different conditions. A simple and excellent breathing exercise, discovered by research academic, Dr Paul Johnson, is to sit up straight, take in a breath, completely filling the lungs, then fully empty them and repeat. Try breathing at 6 breaths per minute. 5 seconds in, 5 seconds out. Allow for a small pause between breaths. This regimen balances the sympathetic and parasympathetic nervous system, as well as improves relaxation and oxygenation. Do this any time you are outside. Fresh, clean air assists healing.

Sunbathing (Heliotherapy)

Every day (privacy permitting) strip naked and take a sun and air bath for a maximum of one hour, when the sun is weak. In 'Nature Cure' centres, they apply organic extra virgin coconut oil to leg ulcers, varicose veins and skin conditions, like eczema and psoriasis, with excellent results. You can also use organic Sesame oil (from black seeds). If you cannot remove your clothes, then sunbathe and apply oil to bare legs. Do not use sun creams, they are toxic. DO NOT BURN.

Sesame Oil

Sesame oil is immensely popular in India. It is a favourite oil for massage, as it penetrates the skin easily, nourishing and detoxifying even the deepest tissue layers. Used regularly, sesame oil is wonderful for reducing stress and tension, nourishing the nervous system and preventing nervous disorders, relieving fatigue and insomnia, while promoting strength and vitality. Regular oiling of the skin restores moisture to the skin, keeping it soft, flexible and young looking. It also lubricates the body internally, particularly the joints and bowels, and eases symptoms of dryness such as irritating coughs, cracking joints and hard stools. Sesame oil massage helps calm babies, lulls them to sleep and improves growth of the brain and the nervous system. Its antioxidants slow the aging process and promote longevity.

Massage and Oil

Massage oils and wet heat help loosen and liquefy toxins in the skin and blood (called the outer disease pathway), dislodging and removing the heavy, sticky toxins from the smallest channels. Thus, toxins begin to drain from the central disease pathway (deeper tissues) and start to flow into the GI tract. Secretions are also activated, enabling easier transport of toxins and wastes as they return to the GI tract for elimination. Oil lubricates and protects tissues from damage, as toxins return to the GI tract. Finally, since Vata (air) is responsible for movement, oil lubrication restores proper Vata functioning, allowing for proper flowing of wastes and toxins to their removal sites. Classical oils to use are Sesame Oil and Castor Oil. Oils can be infused with herbs but this is not required for a DIY program.

Reflexology

Having an expert massage your lower legs and feet is a real treat. An authentic Reflexology session can identify problems in the body and is extremely relaxing except where gout and arthritis exist. Some practitioners use strong pressure to break up crystalline formations. This can be painful but is beneficial. The less painful option is to dissolve crystal formation by alkalyzing the tissues.

Bowel Cleansing

Flushing the bowels at the start of a cleanse, then again during a cleanse, is recommended. Flush the entire gastro-intestinal tract by drinking 1.5-2lts of salt water, within 40 minutes. After 7am is recommended. Most people manage a salt water flush without difficulty. However, if you are particularly toxic, you may feel a little nauseous and may vomit. If so, good! It will cleanse the stomach. Any nausea clears quickly. Ensure you put in enough salt. Salt alters the specific gravity of water, making the body think it is food (not liquid) and thus, directs the salt water to the bowels, instead of kidneys. Use 1 level tablespoon of sea salt in 2lt clean water. If the salt water does not work the first time, increase the amount of salt. Remember, it can do no harm. If for some reason the salt water cannot be taken, drink a laxative tea, night and morning until bowels are clear.

'Mae West' Retention Enema

The Master Cleanse requires a salt water flush (SWF) each morning. However, some people find drinking salt water difficult. If this is you, start with one SWF, on the first morning, then switch to a daily 'Mae West' enema. This has three ingredients. Organic coffee, sea salt and baking soda, added to 2 litres of clean water. Organic coffee stimulates the liver. Sea Salt is cleansing and mineral-rich. Baking soda softens and alkalizes the water. Some people use Colema boards or special colon-cleansing machines but an enema kit with a 2-litre bag is inexpensive and works just fine. Remember, we are seeking simplicity.

1. Put 2 tablespoons of organic coffee in a percolator or boil in a stainless steel pan, in 8-16oz of water.

2. Once boiled, allow to cool a little, add 1 tablespoon each of sea salt and baking soda (aluminium-free).

3. Top up to 2 lts with clean water. Pour into your enema bag.

4. Empty half the contents of the enema bag into your colon (instructions come with the kit). You will feel the need to evacuate. Go ahead and do so, then empty the remaining coffee, into your colon. Try to retain for 15 minutes. If you feel cramping, take deep breaths, until the cramps ease.

Note: Salt water flushes the whole GI tract, while an enema only flushes the lower part of the colon.

Bentonite Shake

Bentonite & Psyllium mixtures are like taking a broom to intestinal walls. They attract and soak up released toxins as well as pull fecal matter off colon walls. Taking this is important during the initial few days, when levels of circulating toxins are high. I make my own but you can buy Dr Schulze Intestinal Formula #2 from here. (I have no affiliation with providers). Here is what the supplier site says:

Intestinal Formula #2 contains the three most powerful and effective absorbers and neutralizers known: clay, charcoal and pectin.

Our Bentonite Clay will actually absorb up to 40 times its weight in intestinal faecal matter and waste. It also smothers and draws out all types of intestinal parasites. The Activated Willow Charcoal is the greatest absorbing agent for every toxin and poison known. It will absorb and render harmless over 3,000 known drug residues, pesticides, insecticides and just about every harmful chemical known. This is why it is the active ingredient in nearly every water filter made today. Apple Pectin draws numerous harmful substances out of your intestines, especially heavy metals like mercury and lead and carcinogenic radioactive materials.

The addition of Marshmallow Root, along with Psyllium Seed and Flax Seed, makes the formula mucilaginous. Mucilaginous means all the water and herbs can sit in your bowel, soaking against the internal wall of your colon, softening and breaking up old, dried and hardened fecal waste that may have been inside you for years.

It is called a shake because you mix the powder with a small amount of water (or fruit juice), shake it, vigorously, and then drink.

Potassium Broth

Potassium broth will flush your system of unwanted salts and acids while providing a concentrated amount of vitamins and minerals. Potassium broth is also a great immune booster.

Ingredients

4 bulbs garlic

2 large onions - peeled

1 bunch chopped kale

1 stick chopped celery

5 pounds chopped carrots

5 pounds potatoes (peels only)

3 beets with greens (peels only)

4 chopped jalapenos

1 bunch organic parsley

4 quarts distilled water

Fill your pot with the chopped vegetables. Cover with distilled or reverse osmosis water and simmer for 1 hour. Add water as needed to keep vegetables covered. Strain, then refrigerate what is not immediately needed. Spread over 2-3 days.

Additional Routines

Every day take a walk outside in your bare feet and shuffle them in the grass or dirt, even lie down on the earth. Use only natural soaps, shampoos and toothpastes. Never use any deodorants, perfumes, colognes, etc. You may use pure herbal essential oils, if you smell. Wear only natural fibre clothing, cotton, wool and silk. No polyester, nylon or even blends.

Liver & Gallbladder Cleanse

The health of our liver is crucial to long-term health. A congested liver is the root reason behind many modern diseases such as acne, yeast infection, leaky gut, etc. Doctors have found that, in almost all cancer patients, the condition of their liver was extremely poor. A congested liver is ultimately caused by an overload of toxins. As a result, the toxins eventually circulate back into your bloodstream, where they can end up anywhere - joints, brain, heart or other organs. Your kidneys become burdened by the extra workload, which contributes to a vicious cycle. If your colon is clogged as well, the liver has an even tougher time eliminating toxins. A congested liver, like a clogged colon, is caused by a poor diet of refined carbohydrates, hydrogenated fats, preservatives, foods laced with hormones, environmental pollutants, over-use of antibiotics, drugs, and stress.

Cholesterol & Bile

We do not need cholesterol from our diet. The liver produces all the cholesterol we need. The liver also produces bile, a greenish-brown fluid, charged with the significant responsibility of digesting fats. Bile is sent to the gallbladder, where it is concentrated and stored. When you eat, the gallbladder contracts and releases stored bile, where it helps break down fat in your food. If the bile within your gallbladder becomes chemically unbalanced, it can form into hardened particles which eventually form stones.

Gallstones

Many statements are made by alternative practitioners saying a liver and gall bladder flush removes gallstones. Our research shows this is true only for some people, with smaller stones and 'chaff' being ejected. Images of thousands of small green 'stones' seen, online, are formed by the olive oil/lemon juice, flush mixture.

'About 1 in 12 people have gallstones and may be unaware of it. As the stones grow and become more numerous the back pressure on the liver causes it to make less bile. It is also thought to slow the flow of lymphatic fluid. Imagine the situation if your garden hose had marbles in it. Much less water would flow, which in turn would decrease the ability of the hose to squirt out the marbles. With gallstones, much less cholesterol leaves the body, and cholesterol levels may rise. Gallstones, being porous, can pick up all the bacteria, cysts, viruses and parasites passing through the liver. In this way "nests" of infection are formed, forever supplying the body with fresh bacteria and parasite stages. No stomach infection such as ulcers or intestinal bloating can be cured permanently without removing these gallstones from the liver.' - Dr Hulda Clark

Our aim is not primarily to remove gallstones (we are pleased when we don't see any) but to clear the liver and gall bladder of toxins, during and after a fast. Flushes are also undertaken to improve overall health. Some people have experienced relief from allergies, bursitis, back pain and other conditions after a liver flush. More so with repeated flushes. If you don't see any stones, be happy! If you ever get a larger stone, you will know about it. The pain is excruciating.

Toxins & Parasites

Anyone conducting a lengthy fast will have parasites dying off from around day 7, while toxins from the deep tissue cleanse (detox), continue to be eliminated. The liver, being the most important organ of elimination, has to work hard to remove this waste from the body. A liver flush opens up the liver and gall bladder ducts, allowing any parasites including Candida to be eliminated more easily. The free flow of bile from the liver/gall bladder will also prevent new parasite infection.

Is the Flush Safe?

Research and feedback, after thousands of flushes, shows this process to be very safe, with only 1 negative incident in 800 reported. The recipe for the flush is hundreds of years old. It involves drinking Epsom salts, followed by an olive oil and lemon juice mix, before retiring. Some have found drinking this difficult, particularly Epsom Salts, which some find unpleasant. It is easier, mixed with apple or grapefruit juice.

Epsom Salts can trigger diarrhoea but not for everyone, since the bowels are already empty after a week or more of fasting. We want the bowel completely empty for the flush anyway. Expect diarrhoea the following morning, possibly a restless night and maybe a little nausea but this quickly wears off. You already do this flush many times a week without realizing it. Eating fat or protein triggers the gallbladder to squeeze itself empty after about twenty minutes, and the stored bile finishes its trip down the common bile duct to the intestine. All we are doing is triggering the same process but in an optimal way. The difference is your bowels will be fully empty and your bile ducts relaxed, due to the magnesium in the Epsom Salts, which acts as both a laxative and muscle relaxant. Oil triggers the gall bladder to empty itself of bile (and anything else in there). Lemon juice helps move the oil along.

'Cold Sheet' Treatment

The Cold Sheet treatment requires two people and is not for the faint-hearted. How does it work? Thanks to Naturopath, Paul Blake, for this explanation:

'Hi I am Paul Blake, a Naturopath, and the Cold Sheet treatment is one of the steps I did to save myself from prostate cancer. I remember quite clearly the first time I finished it and was resting in bed. My mother and step father were sitting across the room and I felt a surge of heat and a buzzing sound in my ears and said "something is coming". The next thing I knew it was morning and I felt tired but wonderful.

There is a great story that goes with the use of the Cold Sheet Treatment or Hydrotherapy (the use of hot and cold water).

In ancient Europe in a small village during the dead of winter a fever had struck the local people and many had died. One night a man who had this fever thought he would try to make it to the local doctors for treatment. So he set out on foot through the heavy snow to the doctor's house, many miles away. Before long it started to snow then turned into a blizzard. The man, sick and cold, pushed on. Soon, in the dark, he came to a fairly wide stream with a fallen log bridge for crossing. In trying to cross the stream the man slipped, fell into the freezing water and was drenched. As he dragged himself out of the icy water he realized he was going to die before he could make it to the doctor. So he turned around hoping to make it back home to his family and at least see them one last time. He was stumbling and delirious by the time he arrived. They tucked him into bed as best they could, expecting him to die. By the morning he had fully recovered; in fact he had not felt this good in years. Even his lumbago was gone. From then on, whenever the man was sick, he would go back to the stream and throw himself in. Well this story got out and spread across Europe and people everywhere from the common man to Kings and Queens were putting themselves through various forms of icy cold and hot treatments to cure their diseases.

From this experience, Hydrotherapy began and the Cold Sheet Treatment was born. At one time hydrotherapy was taught at all medical universities but it was sadly set aside to be replaced by drug therapy. Fortunately, for you and I, intelligent naturopathic doctors like Dr. John Ray Christopher knew better and held on to the treatment because it worked!'

Purpose

The purpose of the Cold Sheet Treatment is to artificially increase the body's temperature, thereby accelerating the body's immune response. The important thing to remember is to keep well hydrated. A high temperature, in a well-hydrated body, is safe and even healthy. The temperature can rise to 103 or 104 degrees Fahrenheit. However if the body is dehydrated, the body can overheat, causing seizure or damage. Drinking plenty of fluids means drinking until your stomach is full and then drinking some more. As Dr. Christopher would say, "When the tea flows out of your ears, that is enough".

Contraindications: Small children, the very elderly, heart disease or moderate-to-severe hypertensive conditions, extreme weakness and debility. Use your common sense! This procedure unmodified is quite rigorous. If you aren't sure, do not use it.

Instructions

Begin with a cool enema of herbal tea. Red Raspberry or Catnip herbal tea is good. This is designed to cleanse and clear the bowel of loose faecal matter in preparation for step 2 the garlic injection. You may want to evacuate the bowel a couple of times. Each time hold the water in the bowel as long as you can before releasing. Be sure and lubricate the enema tip with oil.

Next use a rectal syringe from the drug store to introduce a garlic solution. In a blender mix 8-10 cloves of fresh garlic in 1 cup of water and 1 cup of apple cider vinegar. Filter out garlic pulp and save for step 4 then put the solution in the syringe. For many this is the most intense part of this procedure. It is very safe, but does burn. Squirt in as much of the solution as you can. Keep the garlic solution in as long as you can, usually about 2 minutes before expelling. Even after expelling it, you will retain enough to do you good. The burning and cramping will subside in a couple of minutes.

Make a tea bag out of a sock and add into it 1oz each of Ginger powder, Yellow Mustard powder and Cayenne Pepper powder. Fill the bath as hot as is tolerable without burning the skin and place the sock tea bag in the water. Before the patient gets in, it is important to coat the genitals with plenty of Vaseline. Put the patient in the bath and begin giving them hot/warm herbal tea to drink. Use yarrow (one of the best diaphoretics) or peppermint or ginger tea. The goal is to drink 6-8 full cups of tea. It is the helpers' job to get as much tea as possible into the patient. If the patient becomes faint or light-headed, place a cold washcloth on the forehead. Cayenne tincture in the mouth will also prevent faintness. If the muscles become rigid, or begin to spasm, use Lobelia tincture orally. Keep the patient in the tub for at least 30 minutes. Usually by 20 minutes they'll be aching to get out but keep them in as long as possible, drinking tea until, as mentioned, it is coming out their ears.

Prepare a double sized cotton sheet (it must be 100% cotton) by soaking it in a sink or tub of water and ice. Use lots of ice. Prepare the patients bed by putting a plastic sheet or lining against the mattress under the bed sheets. When the patient stands up, out of the bath, wrap the ice-cold sheet around him/her. Then escort them to bed, wrapped in the sheet. Tuck them into bed, sheet and all, then cover with natural fibre blankets. Wrap them up in a cosy cocoon with a towel around the head leaving a face opening. Dr. Christopher recommends coating the soles of the feet with a thick garlic paste, then putting socks on the feet before putting them in bed. The paste is made by mixing mashed garlic with Vaseline. You can use the garlic you strained from step two. By lying in the sheet for several hours (preferably overnight), the body will continue to sweat out toxins. Often the sheet will be stained with these toxins. Keep the patient in bed for at least 2-3 hours, preferably all night. Upon arising, sponge off with Apple Cider Vinegar and water (half and half) before taking a shower. This will wipe the toxins off the skin so they won't be reabsorbed during the shower. Give the patient only fruit or vegetable juices and herbal teas, for the next 1 to 3 days, to provide a more thorough cleansing. You should continue taking immune boosting herbs and herbal formula such as Echinacea, Goldenseal, Cats Claw, Immune Boost or Anti-Plague Formula.

Modifications to the Cold Sheet Treatment

There are countless modifications to this procedure. For example with a child, you can simply put them in a warm bath, have them drink some herbal tea, give them an Immune herb, like Echinacea, then tuck them into bed. However, for the full impact and benefit, especially when it is life or death, follow the full procedure (Dr Schulze says not to weaken on the enemas or the cold sheet because it seems too radical).

When to Stop a Fast

Dr. Edward Dewey believed you stop fasting when there is no coating on the tongue. If you check your tongue first thing in the morning, it will have a light coating. This is normal. A heavy or darker coloured coating indicates toxicity within the body. Some people use tongue-scrapers when they brush their teeth, as part of their morning ritual or brush the tongue with a toothbrush. It tickles but it works. (If you need to use a tongue-scraper, it is time to clean your body!) Approximately 48hrs after commencing your detox/fast, the coating on the tongue becomes heavier, as the body cleans and liberates more toxins. You will see, over the course of your fast, the coating becoming lighter. For those who are particularly toxic, this can take upward of 30 days.

The other indicator of when to stop is when you feel well again. While visible Arthritis symptoms can disappear in as little as 10 days, it may need longer to ensure your disease is truly vanquished. Lifestyle changes will ensure symptoms do not return.

Where to Buy Supplements?

At the retreat we source most of our supplies locally, since imports are difficult to get through customs and are expensive. It isn't really necessary to import anything when nature provides all you need, where you live. If you are not sure, one of the first places to start is your local health store. You can also find and purchase what you need, online, such as Dr Schulze online herbal pharmacy.

About Cancer

It is possible someone may attempt to resolve their cancer, based on protocols they read here. I recommend you do not try this yourself, without professional assistance. When tumours start to break down the debris released can make you very ill, even causing death. This tumour material needs to be removed from the body, safely. Coffee enemas are often used, since they assist the liver in detoxification. Additionally, for cancer, I would add proteolytic enzymes and probiotics to my regime. If you recall, this combination cured the 'great great' Dr. Bernard Jensen.

What If I Am Still Sick?

While I believe most conditions can be halted, or reversed, there may be some which stubbornly refuse to improve. As you have read, numerous disorders are linked by experts to fluoride, aluminium or mercury poisoning. The dramatic increase in health disorders in the U.S. should remove any doubt. Specialists working with autism have shown heavy metal detoxification improves autism and sometimes completely reverses it. The key is to get the offending toxin out of your tissues. If you have still not recovered, you can either repeat the 30 day program and see how you feel, or undertake a more focussed Fluoride or Heavy Metal detox. We offer these as Retreats or Online Health Coaching sessions. You can find details at the rear of the book or the relevant page on the website. Or you can try any of the following.

'Magic Bullet' Cures

I previously dismissed 'Magic Bullets' since, unless you know exactly what is the cause of your disease and the precise antidote, you will invariably fail to see results. Yet, when you look at the cures I have suggested, three stand out as 'Magic Bullets'. The first is water. What does it do? It alkalyzes and hydrates (flushes) the tissues and brings more oxygen to the cells.

The second is urine. After suffering greatly, trying everything and spending vast amounts of money over a 30-year period, Martha Cristy was cured of all her diseases, simply by drinking her own urine.

The third is oxygen. According to Ed McCabe, bringing more oxygen to your cells can cure 99% of disease. (By the way, juice and water-fasting both increase oxygenation of cells.)

"All disease is caused by some sort of blockage. Whether it's blocked blood, lymph, oxygen, nutrition, nerve impulse, emotional energy, spiritual energy, or even what the Chinese, Japanese or Indians refer to as Chi, Ki, or Prana. When an area of the body gets blocked, it gets sick. It's that simple."

Dr. Richard Schulze

Placebo vs Nocebo

You have probably heard of the 'Placebo effect'. This is where the power of your own belief heals you. The Doctor gives you some sugar pills, tells you it is medicine and you get well. The Placebo effect is accepted by the Medical profession even though not fully understood.

When it comes to the power of positive thinking or 'mind over matter', Doctors tend to describe the idea as 'New Age twaddle,' or the latest scornful label, 'woo'. This is curious when there are many officially recorded incidents of patients being healed from 'incurable' diseases. Doctors call these 'Spontaneous Remissions' and there is a database for them. They are better described as 'Radical Remissions' since when you investigate them, there is nothing spontaneous about them at all. Individuals play a full part in their own cure.

The Spontaneous Remission Project has been put together by the Institute of Noetic Sciences and has over 3500 case studies published in the medical literature about people who experienced spontaneous remissions from seemingly 'incurable diseases.' Most of the case studies involved people with Stage 4 cancers who either declined conventional treatment or were given treatment deemed by doctors to be inadequate for cure. There are also case studies of those who recovered from other 'incurable' diseases, such as heart failure, autoimmune disease and HIV.

Dr Lissa Rankin, an American physician who has investigated self-healing, has this on her website:

'Dr. Lissa Rankin was a skeptical physician, trained in evidence-based academic medicine and raised by a closed-minded physician father. But after witnessing patients who declined conventional medical treatment, only to experience spontaneous remissions from seemingly "incurable" illnesses, she couldn't deny the possibility patients might hold within them the power to heal themselves. Her curiosity led her to dig deep into the medical literature to scientifically prove the mind can heal the body. Her search uncovered not only proof you can heal yourself, but also the shocking physiological mechanisms of how emotions like fear, loneliness, pessimism, and depression can make the body sick, while love, intimate connection, optimism, and faith can cure you'.

Dr Rankin reports approximately 30% of patients, given placebo, will heal 'spontaneously'. This, of course, is good news because it confirms positive thinking influences our ability to heal and should be part of any healing protocol.

Take care, though. The 'Placebo Effect' has its alter ego. This is called the 'Nocebo Effect'. What happens when someone is given a Cancer or AIDS diagnosis? They are so convinced they are going to die you can see the will to live drain out of them. I have met people like this. A friend has advanced Emphysema and is convinced he is going to die. Information from me changed his mind but he took a lot of convincing. Dr Rankin has found cases where patients have been informed of side effects of a drug and they have gone on to manifest those same side effects, even though they had been given sugar pills. Could this be the real reason Doctors rarely tell you of the risks? I doubt it but it's nice to think so.

So there you have it.

BELIEVING you will die or sicken can CAUSE you to die or sicken.

BELIEVING you will heal and will live can CAUSE you to heal and live.

Watch what you believe. Your cells are listening!

"80% of my patients were well just after doing my thorough bowel cleansing program"

Richard Schulze

Nature Cure

Naturopathy believes in two things.

1.   We fall ill when we violate the laws of nature.

2.   All healing powers lie within the body.

This is a different concept to mainstream medicine, particularly since the 1800's and the advent of 'heroic medicine'. This is when regular Doctors made Nature redundant and decided they could do a better (heroic) job of it. An example of this attitude is the teaching of medical professor Benjamin Rush, who advised his students,

"Always treat nature in a sick room as you would a noisy dog or cat. Drive her out the door and lock it upon her".

Allopathic Doctors' belief in the superiority of their methods has remained undiminished, even in the face of staggering failure. Disease is widespread and growing and the allopathic system of medicine is contributing to, rather than, reducing it. They may quote him but Hippocrates would instantly disown the doctors of today. Hippocrates believed in natural healing, as did the founder of the Thomsonian School of Healing, Samuel Thomson, from which sprung Dr Richard Schulze. The fundamental 'vitalistic' principles of natural healing had not changed for a thousand years when the 'Mechanists' decided to reduce the body to its physical and chemical constituents.

'Nature Cure' is a very simple system, based on common sense. Support the body's own efforts to heal. Use cleansing, diet, herbs, exercise, sunlight, hydrotherapy, stress reduction and, where people are open, spiritual power. In India I observed patients who had been rejected by the hospitals and sent home to die, completely recover at Nature Cure Centres. This system might have been more widely taken up had it not been as simple as it is. Unfortunately, the public is more impressed by the complex and mysterious. Scientific, technically-brilliant, mechanistic Doctors are too aloof, patriarchal and condescending to consider giving patients a hug, a mug of herbal tea, and a massage.

Ayurveda

What is Ayurveda? The name itself means 'Science of Life' or 'Knowledge of Life'. Its origins are said to go back 3-5000 years. The oldest system of lifestyle and medicine in the world. Ayurveda is a comprehensive, eco-friendly, holistic, 'Mind-Body' system of living, which addresses the whole person. Ayurveda incorporates healing, using natural, non-toxic, non-invasive techniques, to restore body, mind and spirit. These include the classic naturopathic components: nutrition, exercise, detoxification, bodywork, herbs, emotional healing and stress reduction.

In India, today's Ayurveda has two strands, ancient and modern, both of which are fully supported by the Indian Government and the World Health Organization. Approximately two-thirds of India's rural people, who comprise 70 percent of the population, use Ayurveda for their primary health care needs. In India, Ayurvedic Doctors train as conventional medical Doctors, then go on to qualify in Ayurveda. Some specialize even further. In the West we are most familiar with the exercise part of Ayurveda, Hatha Yoga. Yoga is a 'mind-body' system. Qi Gong and Tai Chi are similar 'mind-body' systems. Yoga is an integral part of Ayurveda, designed to strengthen and relax the body. In the west, although we have cherry-picked Hatha Yoga and ignored the rest of the Ayurvedic System, it is still highly beneficial. The ancients did not wish the body to interfere with meditation. You cannot meditate if you cannot sit still! If you have practiced Yoga for any length of time, you understand how beneficial it is in strengthening and calming the body.

Hatha Yoga

In the West, Hatha Yoga is more a physical exercise program than a method of improving self-awareness and achieving union. Bodies are encouraged into various positions, allied to their breathing, followed by deep relaxation. There are many schools of Yoga. Iyengar, Sivananda, Kundalini, Ashtanga, Kriya and more. While only a minor part of the Ayurvedic system, Hatha Yoga is suitable for everyone, takes up very little space, does not need any equipment and once you grasp the basic moves, you can practice at home, at no cost. No need to pound the pavements and stress those weight-bearing joints. Hatha Yoga relaxes and strengthens the body, which calms the mind. A super introduction to Yoga is to find a 'Laughter Yoga' class. It is not really Yoga but is great fun all the same. Laughter is the BEST medicine!

Raja Yoga

Less well known, Raja Yoga focuses on developing mastery over the mind. It means the Royal Path. Raja Yoga has techniques for controlling our desires, improving concentration, bringing us back to our true nature and achieving peace of mind. Raja Yoga sees no need for physical postures, instead concentrating on calming the mind, which relaxes the body. In the Brahma Kumaris version I practiced, we would sit on a comfy chair or sofa. No need to sit with rigid spines. Brahma Kumaris, is a world-wide organization, affiliated to the United Nations. They offer Positive Thinking and Stress Management courses for individuals and corporations, based on Raja Yoga. These courses strip out much of the Indian terminology, which many westerners find off-putting. If you can find a branch near you, I highly recommend attending a class. Some people regard this organization as cult-like, so beware.

Raja Yoga. The mind affects the body. Hatha Yoga. The body affects the mind. One works from the outside-in. The other from the inside-out. You see? You can practice them separately but, in my experience, learn more and achieve better results practicing them together.

'Ice-Cream for the Mind'

A useful and popular mental relaxation and concentration exercise is called Transcendental Meditation (TM). This technique, introduced to the West from India in the late 50s, involves the repetition of one word, a mantra, which you practice for 10-20 minutes, twice a day. It is impossible to quiet an unruly mind by trying NOT to think. Struggle is force and all you will find is the mind becomes more agitated if you attempt to subdue it. The opposite of what you are seeking. The ancients learned, mechanically repeating a word (mantra), or phrase, has a settling effect on the mind. If you practice correctly, there is no effort. No struggle. The cost of joining a TM program can be high. Perversely, when you give techniques like this away, free, people tend not to apply them. High prices motivate people to do the practice, since they do not wish to 'waste their money' or they perceive a higher value. I saw this in action with my wife (apologies to her for sharing!). I once worked for a cosmetics company. One day I went down to the production line and filled a large unmarked bottle with an Estee Lauder face cream, worth hundreds of pounds. I presented this to my wife, rather unceremoniously (plonked it on the kitchen table). She never used it. There was no pretty packaging or expensive outlay.

Techniques such as TM are universal knowledge and should be accessible to all, not just to those who can afford it, which is why I offer them to our Retreat guests. Contrary to popular belief, the TM mantras are neither new nor unique. They are ancient and well known in Ayurveda. Just not in the West. There are subtle differences between mantras, so you need to select (or be given) the mantra to suit your need, your 'Chakra' (See appendix) and your Constitutional Type.

An old Cherokee is teaching his grandson about life. "A fight is going on inside me," he said to the boy. "It is a terrible fight and it is between two wolves. One is evil – he is anger, envy, sorrow, regret, greed, arrogance, self-pity, guilt, resentment, inferiority, lies, false pride, superiority, and ego." He continued, "The other is good – he is joy, peace, love, hope, serenity, humility, kindness, benevolence, empathy, generosity, truth, compassion, and faith. The same fight is going on inside you – and inside every other person, too." The grandson thought about it for a minute and then asked his grandfather, "Which wolf will win?" The old Cherokee simply replied, "The one you feed the most."

Who Am I?

I am an ordinary man, with a passion for truth and compassion for others. A career in the military and love of travel has seen me spend much of my life travelling and living abroad. Today, I have a family and am settled, although kept busy with retreats, online health coaching and writing books like this. Health-wise, I learned 'auto-didactically' (mostly self-taught), with twenty five years of investigating alternative and natural methods of healing, trying to cure my own chronic and degenerative disorders. Conventional medicine only damaged me until the penny eventually dropped and I FIRED MY DOCTOR.

I am not an academic, professional author or licenced medical practitioner. I provide knowledge and support to those who wish to help themselves. I write as a consumer and Natural Healing advocate. Health matters fascinate me and there is always more to learn. During the last two and a half decades I have become versed in various healing techniques, both their theory and practical application. The Thomsonian School of Healing, Gandhi's 'Nature Cure', Ayurveda and more. The latter two I studied in Kerala, India, the 'Home of Ayurveda'. I teach Yoga as therapy along with several meditation techniques, can design nutritional healing plans and give a passable Thai Massage. I spent 2 years in a Raja Yoga Retreat, then went on to learn EFT+NLP, 'Breaking The Chains', juice and water fasting, Reiki, oxygen therapies and herbalism. Everything that is needed in an Holistic Healing Toolkit. Living several years next to a Healing Retreat, where visiting practitioners would hold regular workshops, considerably expanded my knowledge. As did a long period of experimentation with esoteric-minded friends, learning about local herbs and how to prepare them. We practiced breathing exercises, bodywork, hydrotherapy, organic gardening, psychological and emotional healing and more. Pretty much the whole gamut of natural therapies.

With every new technique I encountered, I kept an open mind and did not allow anyone else to decide for me who was a charlatan and what was 'quackery' (the Health Industry's code word for competition). This was a world apart from my previous attitude, which had absolute faith and acceptance of modern medicine because it has been 'scientifically proven' and everything unproven must, therefore, be bogus. A little investigation soon shatters that myth. Today, whenever the corporate media run hit-pieces, going after alternative practices or practitioners, I no longer nod in approval but become intensely interested. "Why are they working so hard to demonize this person, supplement or technique?" It is surprising what you learn once you investigate.

On the psycho/emotional side my lengthy struggle with chronic anxiety, panic disorder and 'burn-out', gave me valuable insights into how ineffective Psychiatry is and how depression, anger, anxiety and addictions can be resolved without resorting to harmful chemistry or taking an electric drill to the side of my skull. Internet 'bashers', bent on mischief, demand to know my medical qualifications, as if only the qualified can comment on health matters. This is just silliness. For most people, recovering their health is simple because the causes of their disorders are simple. If you believe in true freedom, as opposed to medical dictatorship, everyone has a right, even a moral imperative, to take care of themselves and others.

I am sometimes asked, "You know a lot about health. Why not qualify?" A reasonable question but in what? If conventional medicine is unable to cure chronic degenerative disorders, what does that say about its qualifications? According to the literature, around 100 years ago, allopathic medical education was taken over by the Rockefeller and Carnegie Corporations and JP Morgan bank. This powerful alliance skewed health education toward pharmaceutical medicines derived from crude oil. Improvement was certainly needed at the time. The profession endured a poor reputation. Medical Degrees could be easily purchased through the mail or obtained with the minimum of training. Today, Doctors medical education is high quality, if narrow. In disease management and pharmaceutical medicine, they excel. In emergency and acute disorders, they excel. Unfortunately, where it matters, in nutrition, prevention, treating the whole person, addressing underlying cause and using non-toxic, non-invasive methods of healing, they are lost at sea in their genomes and minimalist specializations.

It is hardly the Doctor's fault if their education is narrow and focus misdirected. The medical profession has been expertly trained to look in the wrong direction. President Obama's 'Precision Medicine Initiative' the latest example. Here is a message for policy-makers. Forget genetics, which is responsible for only 1% of disorders. Get out in the street and start dealing with the real killers in our midst. Poverty, violence, lack of education and opportunity, junk food, polluted relationships, polluted environment, corrupt media and politics, endless wars, social deprivation and injustice.

Of what use is a qualification if not backed by ethical behaviour? In recent years, the Health Industry in America has abandoned ethics. 95% of Doctors have taken 'inducements' from drug companies - free meals, tickets to the basketball game, seminars in the Bahamas and so on - to encourage them to prescribe the latest 'blockbuster' drug, rather than cheaper, more effective medicines, whose patents have expired. Lead Doctors, some earning millions, are shamelessly on drug companies' payroll.

What about Alternative Medicine? Well, schools such as Bastyr University in the U.S. have an interesting Ayurvedic Master of Science program, covering medical Sanskrit, psychology, yoga, pathology, herbal therapies and nutrition. I've been studying Ayurveda since before it became fashionable. A Doctor of Naturopathy is another possibility but I am getting a bit long in the tooth to go back to school. Ethical questions surround alternative practitioners, too. Many have entered the health field to do one thing and one thing only. Make money. An army of practitioners has qualified, perhaps via Correspondence Course or night school, in minor therapies like massage, Reiki, EFT and so on. This allows them to make a living. However, ask them where the gall bladder or spleen is and they have no idea. They know nothing of Anatomy and Physiology. It may not be so necessary for them to know but you can understand why conventional medicine is dismissive. How can someone doing a 2-day Reiki course compare to a Doctor who has spent 12 years in high-level study? Why is it NOT that necessary for Alternative practitioners to learn Anatomy and Physiology? Well, their particular discipline may not require it. Do I need to know the inner workings of my car's engine to give it the right fuel? Of course not. The Medical profession's arrogance is summed up nicely in this poem from the late 1800's:

"Tis nature that does it – but what right has she

To be round curing people without a degree?

A man to be cured without sending for me!

Without sending for any right licenced M.D.!!

It's unscientific, irregular, mean----

The shamefulest thing that ever was seen!"

Mad Dads' and 'Crazy Mums'

25 years ago, after a sustained period of high stress, I broke down. Physically, psychologically, emotionally and spiritually. Ten years later I came within a whisker of breaking down again. I was 'burnt-out', suffering chronic anxiety, panic attacks and living in a 'dark pit of despair' (if you have ever been 'in the pit', you will understand).

What could have upset my mind to the extent I needed to, off and on, spend 3 ½ years on anti-depressants, just to sleep? The possibilities seem endless. A trigger but not the cause was the premature birth and struggle for life of my daughter. I spent years trying to understand what happened to me and why I was unable to bounce back. Having seen Doctors, Psychiatrists and therapists of every stripe, I began to build a picture. Each interaction, another brick in my wall of understanding. 20 different psychiatrists would give me 20 different reasons why I was depressed and anxious, all of which sounded plausible. The solution, though, always came back to chemistry. The need to correct a supposed 'imbalance in the brain'. I didn't understand then, but certainly do now, the poisonous compounds they gave me were not correcting imbalances. They were creating them.

Delving into a troubled mind is like falling down the rabbit-hole in Alice in Wonderland. You enter a chaotic landscape, filled with imaginary creatures that seem all too real. After following umpteen different trails, I was completely lost. Was I really sexually abused as a child? Was some dark family secret, from generations ago, pervading my present psyche? Did my inner child need a hug? Was my previously dormant soul awakening? My self-esteem or self-confidence, too low? Was it Social Anxiety Disorder? Post-Traumatic Stress Disorder? Generalized Anxiety Disorder? Gulf War Syndrome? Mercury or radiation-poisoning? Adrenal Exhaustion (absolutely)? Were the anti-depressants, causing the very anxiety and suicidal thoughts they claim to relieve? (curious how so many drugs do this).

I was dead to all feeling, doped mostly with Seroxat, an SSRI class of psychiatric drug, containing Fluoride. Other brand names in this class are:

Citalopram (Celexa)

Escitalopram (Lexapro)

Fluoxetine (Prozac)

Paroxetine (Paxil, Pexeva)

Sertraline (Zoloft)

If fluoride can have such a numbing effect on my brain I can understand the controversy over dumping millions of tons of it into our water supply and adding it to toothpaste and a myriad of other products. That aside, I was initially grateful for the sleep it afforded me. Until the side effects began to manifest, which the Doctor somehow forgot to mention. Addiction, permanent brain changes, chronic fatigue, suicidal thoughts and sexual dysfunction. My once-vital sex life deteriorated and has been... ahem... up and down ever since. "Thanks, Doc."

After years of getting nowhere, I finally wrapped all the theories up in a large black bag labelled 'Psychobabble' and tossed them in the bin. Later, I came to a startling realization. It was NONE of those things. All these apparent causes disappeared in a puff of smoke once I identified and corrected the underlying physical cause. Nutritional deficiency. Something had wiped out the microvilli in my intestines (which absorb nutrients from food). Modern diets are already nutritionally deficient but, for me, the problem was compounded because I was unable to extract nutrients, even if present. Chronic gut inflammation contributed to the Alternative practitioners' favourite 'goto', Leaky Gut. This is where the lining of the gut becomes porous, allowing undigested food particles and proteins to pass through the intestinal wall into the bloodstream, eventually lodging in the joints or elsewhere. Hello, arthritis. Support for Hippocrates when he said, "All disease begins in the gut".

A common side effect of malnutrition is depression and anxiety, since the brain is also starved of nutrients. Symptoms manifest in the mind, so we are referred to psychiatry, which is armed and ready to club it into submission with an array of toxic poisons. Of all the experts I saw over the years, psychiatrists, psychotherapists, hypnotherapists, etc.., not one considered there may be a physical cause to my psychological problems. Not one realized important nutrients, which provide resilience to stress, had been gobbled up by life events, until my nutrient bank was empty. I was not deficient in Prozac or Valium or Beta-blockers or Seroxat but B1, B2, B3, B5, B12, Folic Acid, fats and oils. My adrenal glands (which produce stress hormones) were worn out from spending too many years in 'fight or fight' mode. I was not so much a 'Mad Dad' but a starving dad. Nor was I alone. 18 million adults in the U.S. suffer anxiety disorders. 350 million people around the world suffer depression, more women than men. Could it be that, for most of these millions, the root of their problem lies not on the psychiatrist's couch but on the dinner table?

'**Nutritional Neuroscience**' is starting to shed light on this:

'...essential vitamins, minerals, and omega-3 fatty acids are often deficient in the general population in America and other developed countries; and are exceptionally deficient in patients suffering from mental disorders. Studies have shown daily supplements of vital nutrients often effectively reduce patients' symptoms.'

One healing science using nutrient supplementation is 'Orthomolecular Medicine', which means healing through nutrition. Advocates like the witty and insightful author Andrew Saul, provide numerous examples where Niacin has worked wonders on psychiatric patients. Alone, it would not have resolved my Celiac Disease but it may have eased anxiety and panic attacks. Niacin was the solution offered by the Naturopath who said he could have cured me in 3 days.

Chronic stress and its effects on long term health are a recognized problem. In warfare, 30% of servicemen will experience some kind of stress disorder. If I could study them, I am sure I would find most would be 'Air' Types (See Appendix). This Constitutional Type naturally tend toward nervous disorders. Chronic stress can seriously threaten physical and emotional well-being, triggering psychosomatic illness. There exists a huge lack of understanding, by society, of what stress is, its causes, how pressure builds up over time and how it can be dealt with, effectively, at an early stage.

Having taken the decision to escape the pressure I was under (an action I should have taken a decade before), I set about restoring my psychological and physical health. My joints were painful, there were seasonal allergies and over the years, heart disease (chest pain), fibromyalgia, inflammatory bowel disease, hypoglycaemia, enlarged prostate and inguinal hernias. My hands trembled, I bruised easily, was constantly fatigued and underweight. Tension headaches, foggy thinking, poor concentration and memory were constant companions. The physical ailments were almost all due to prolonged tension. Tension in the mind causes tension in the body and vice-versa. When muscles and tendons are tight, blood flow, nerve flow, lymph flow and vital energy are restricted or blocked. The constant circulation of stress hormones upsets the digestive system, along with the acid/alkaline balance. Stress is devastating to the whole person.

Abandoning Ship

After 'The Peace That Passeth All Understanding' had ebbed away, my stress returned and my marriage started to fail. What was the answer from the orthodoxy? Chemicals. Antibiotics. Painkillers. Anti-inflammatories. Anti-histamines. Beta-blockers. Anti-anxiety medication. Muscle-relaxants. Chemical after chemical. No concern for root cause. Only management of symptoms, with a sustained assault on my liver. After years of this, I understood. No Doctor was going to CURE me. How could they? They had no real idea what was wrong with me. With my joints increasingly painful, I had no choice in the matter. In my anxiety-filled state, visions of an early grave, if I did not act, appalled me. I had to get away.

The unsympathetic portray my escape as 'running away'. Evidence of a lack of moral character. They believe we all have crises at some point in our lives and should simply shrug them off, pick ourselves up and carry on. As if this wasn't blindingly obvious. Of course, I and my loved ones wished all had been well. Had the events which tipped me into crisis not taken place, my life and the lives of those around me might have been very different. Yet, it was not to be. Whatever the effect on others of my leaving, I was of no use to anyone as a suicide statistic. Which leads me to make a plea. If you are ever faced with an individual who is stressed or suicidal, try not to condemn them. You have no idea what they may have been through. They do not need your condemnation. Along with physical, emotional and psychological support, sufferers need patience, tolerance and understanding. They also, as I discovered, require proper nutrition. Show some compassion. Next time it could be you.

I am not expecting you to do as I did. You may not have the time, money, or opportunity to retreat into the wilderness. BUT if you are suicidal or dying from disease, you must do whatever it takes to get well. I jumped on a motorbike, left everything behind, crossed the English Channel, rode over the Alps, travelled down through the Pyrenees, on into Portugal, where I landed on a barren hillside in the Algarve. After a year of isolation, in a derelict farmhouse, working on myself with Hatha Yoga, I spent 2 years in a Raja Yoga retreat, learning how the mind works and mastering techniques for bringing it under control. No need for me to remain at the mercy of my mind. I could become its Master!

The flavour of Raja Yoga I embraced, encouraged purity. Pure thoughts, right action, pure food, celibacy and knowledge of how to live one's life. Combined with meditation, I experienced a noticeable improvement. Observers would remark how brilliant and clear my eyes were (the 'Windows to the Soul'). My body certainly felt clean. Yet, for all its benefits, my recovery wasn't complete. I was 80% better. Good but not good enough.

Living a life of celibacy was easy after the trauma of separation and divorce. The last thing I wanted or needed was another relationship. But as time passed and my vitality and optimism returned, so did the twinkle in my eye. Repressing one's natural urges isn't wise, as many an unfrocked Priest has discovered. The sexual urge is one of the strongest instincts in man. While I could have spent the rest of my life as an ascetic and would probably have been happier in a retreat than living in the 'normal' world. I knew, instinctively, it was time to leave.

Those years of meditation had shown me one thing. How difficult it is to settle the western mind. Our nervous systems are so over-stimulated by TV, technology, drugs, medications, the workings of our mind and the constant gratification of the senses, we cannot sit still for five minutes. We have lost the ability to relax. I have witnessed many give up on meditation before it had a chance to demonstrate its benefits. Defeated by their bodies. This is why Hatha Yoga is an integral part of the Ayurvedic/Yoga system. The body needs to be trained to relax and concentrate before meditation is possible. If you find yourself fidgeting too much don't be discouraged. Work on relaxing your body.

Another preparatory step, before meditation is possible, is concentration. Which is why some disciplines focus on a single object. Either a point of light, an image, or a mantra.

The Long Dark Night of the Soul

This period in my life was, without doubt, the most difficult I have ever had to endure. A lengthy and profound absence of light and hope. Breaking down. In a pit of despair. Profoundly alone. Suicide the only way out. Imagine only getting one hour's sleep per night. The pressure in your head so intense you want to drill a hole in your temple to relieve it. Fear and anxiety so overwhelming your heart pounds and you feel like you cannot breathe. That you are dying or 'going crazy'. Imagine experiencing this, not for minutes or hours but months. Today, if you were to ask me about this period, I would call it a blessing. The prelude to re-birth. A stage I had to go through to transform from the old to the new.

Cancer survivors sometimes say their cancer was the best thing that ever happened to them because it forced them to take a good look at themselves. To alter their disease-inducing lifestyles; re-examine their values and beliefs; emerge from their disease with an improved outlook on life. I am certainly not unique. 10% of people go through a major crisis at some point in their lives, asking the same profound questions.

"Who am I?"

"What is my purpose in life?"

"Is this all there is?"

Was I just an entry in a government and corporate database, branded and tracked, from birth by my social security number? Estimated by corporate bean-counters to be worth $1,000,000 in potential profits as soon as I exit the womb. A conditioned drone, living a pre-determined, material existence, until death or taxes finish me. Surely my value as a human being was worth more than a pointless vote every four years to decide which set of white-collar criminals get to plunder the public purse? We are much more than this. Organized religion may have been undermined by its leaders and a concerted campaign by the media and Hollywood to destroy it but I would rather be seen as a wonderful, unique creation of 'God', a place reserved for me at his right hand, than a 'profit opportunity' for the already wealthy, stripped of all dignity, my remaining assets pounced on in the last two years of life.

Few of my military colleagues will live to collect their pensions. I have heard the official figure is as low as 11%. My father, a former soldier, died the day his first pension cheque hit his bank account. He was 55. A father-in-law died, an empty whisky bottle in his hand, at 49. A lawyer friend, 50, when his heart gave out. Today I am grateful for each day. Sickness or suicide came very close to finishing me.

I Fired My Doctor!

My GP, while sympathetic, had little time to do anything other than prescribe anti-depressants. Psychiatrists and psychiatric nurses, in the UK, commendably introduced me to non-drug approaches, such as relaxation training and stress management. Yet, so fried was my mind, I was forced to remain on the drugs.

Whether it is immediately obvious, or becomes clear over time, firing your Doctor is a necessary step to healing. For reasons, relating to my children, it was 10 years before I took this step. Time can be saved by asking your Doctor a simple question, "CAN YOU CURE ME?" By that, I mean can he or she create the conditions which will allow your body and mind to heal? If the answer is "No", walk out. Unless you are content with temporary relief of symptoms. Some are.

The first step was to remove myself from the pressures I was under. Then find space and time to come off the anti-depressants. After abandoning my comfortable home in England, I landed on a Portuguese hillside in the Algarve, living in a dilapidated farmhouse, with no running water and few amenities. Like something from a film set, my room was a stark space, with white plaster falling off stone walls. A single bed, wooden chair and bare bulb, providing dim light. I showered using cold water from a bucket. That was it. Nothing else. No TV. No radio. No computer. No phone. No ornamental clutter, requiring shelves and then more shelves, to accommodate it all. The perfect sanctuary for an ascetic monk and my wrecked nervous system. The lack of visual and aural stimulation may seem like purgatory to some but it was heaven to me.

Each day I would walk the lavender-covered hills, with not a soul to be seen for miles. I could not run, my arthritic knees hurt. So Yoga was the chosen exercise. For five hours a day I practiced. Three hours in the morning and two in the afternoon. I adopted a vegan diet, breathed in unpolluted air, sunbathed, read self-help books like this and learned as much as I could about mental and physical health. Eventually my efforts started to bear fruit. My nerves began to settle, mind began to calm and despite an alarming 3 months (I failed the first time) coming off the Seroxat, I started to feel somewhat human again. Why had I failed on the first attempt? When I stopped the tablets, a frightening wave of anxiety and suicidal thinking hit me. No wonder so many remain on these drugs for life. It does not surprise me to read many of those involved in school shootings were on anti-depressants.

It had taken a year to reach this stage. While I was over the worst, I wasn't cured. The winters in Portugal were a challenge. Properties were not built for cold weather and during weeks of rainfall, my arthritis flared. The vegan diet, supposedly the best diet for health, left me tired and undernourished. I was still carrying around a deep, unresolved fear. I would end up like my mother. What did my mother have to do with it? Plenty. All the mental and physical symptoms, my mother also had before me. She endured a painful and prolonged death. Today there is a lot of talk about genetics. Doctors may say "It's genetic" when they don't know what is wrong with us. Scripture informs us the 'Sins of the fathers shall be visited upon the children'. Did that mean in the form of disease? 'Bad blood' or weak semen? Had I been poisoned by chemicals in my mother's breast milk? What about her mercury fillings or vaccines? Could they have injured me in the womb? Was some genetic defect passed on to me? Had I been injured by mercury or fluoride or aluminium? If so, why not my brother and sister? I often see children develop the same disorders as their parents, by adopting the same toxic lifestyle and disease-inducing diet. Were my mother and I intolerant of, or sickened by, the same foods? There were some indicators of food sensitivity from an early age. A runny nose after eating porridge (oatmeal). Mouth ulcers after eating biscuits or popcorn. When young, you pay little attention.

My mother struggled most of her adult life with illness. Some real. Some imagined. I am not sure which was which. She embraced hypochondria like a warm blanket. Sickness kept my social father home and brought her the attention she appeared to crave. After many years of feigning illness, we children were drained of all sympathy. Eventually she developed full blown Rheumatoid Arthritis, the treatment of which eventually killed her. Her last two years of life were a torment, with constant pain and botched operations. She learned about 'complications' the hard way. After one trip to the Intensive Care Unit due to a surgical error (her bowel was perforated), she was left wearing a colostomy bag for life. You could feel her humiliation and sadness. This was the future I was facing. Orthodox treatments for Rheumatoid Arthritis have barely changed. A painful and prolonged death. An overdose of morphine eventually put my mother out of her misery, adding weight to Moliere's words, uttered hundreds of years ago... 'Nearly all men die of their remedies and not of their illnesses.'

Shopping at the Alternative Healing Bazaar

For many years after firing my Doctor, I dived into the murky waters of Alternative practitioners and their techniques. Acupuncture, Cranial Osteopathy, Chiropractic, Traditional Chinese Medicine, Ayurveda (both ancient and modern), Thai Traditional Medicine, Homeopaths, Osteopaths, Naturopaths, Astrologers, Faith Healers, Mediums, Reiki Masters, Herbalists, Yogis, Hypnotherapists, Shamen, Sufi and Christian Priests. Emotional and Spiritual Healers. Add to this the endless number of 'Wonder Cures' available online, all major credit cards accepted. I was a Grasshopper. Hopping from treatment to treatment, never staying with one method long enough to realize significant benefit. Like prospecting for oil. I sank lots of wells but never struck oil because I never drilled deep enough. Unconsciously always seeking the quick fix. I became well versed in alternatives and could impress everyone with my knowledge. On my travels I met many, like me, shoppers at the Alternative Healing Bazaar. Knowledgeable and not cured.

What is less impressive and you may have met them, are those who do not practice what they preach. I know an Ayurvedic Doctor who teaches Yoga and meditation and offers healthy Indian food. Yet his stomach expands every time I see him. If you are extolling the virtues of juice fasting and how wonderful it is for your skin, it is no use your own skin looking like orange peel. If you are selling the benefits of balancing the autonomic nervous system, it does not look good if you cannot sit still. Similarly, if you are marketing weight loss products, it doesn't look good carrying around a distended belly. There are examples everywhere I look, such as Monks in certain parts of Asia, smoking.

Likewise, modern Doctors and Psychiatrists. They help others but do not look after themselves. If you are a psychiatrist it doesn't help your credibility if you look like an axe-murderer. I look at some and Jesus instruction springs to mind, "Physician. Heal thyself." It is not they were not genuine, or their methods did not have the potential to cure. I am confident each wished to help and had something useful to offer.

Whatever the therapy, or degree of success, at least they operated in accordance with Hippocrates instruction: "First Do No Harm".

'Doctor Brain'

India is not just synonymous with curries and population growth. It is considered the cradle of civilization. Much of our medical knowledge came from the ancient gurus and yogis of India. The ancients had a great understanding of mind and body. They understood, thousands of years ago, what western Doctors and Psychiatrists fail to grasp. You cannot separate head from body and expect people to get better. So, it was to the ancients I turned when my mind was in turmoil. In particular, the healing systems known as Ayurveda and Nature Cure.

Ayurveda is much more than the two strands of Yoga, Hatha and Raja. It incorporates a set of values and morals, involves nutrition, herbs, detoxification of The Five Layers, as well as astrological components. It is an holistic system, based on what Constitutional Type you may be. There are a number of methods of typing people flying around but I have found the Ayurvedic Theory of Elements... Earth, Air, Fire, Water and Ether... to fit reasonably accurately. (See Appendix for more on Ayurvedic Constitutional Types).

What was I going to do about my Arthritis? In conventional western medicine, there is no cure. In fact, as my mother found out, the treatment can be worse than the disease. It still is. I saw little point in going down the conventional medical route. In 2004, hearing good things about Ayurveda, I decided to try it. So, it was off to Kerala, the 'Home of Ayurveda' in India, with a friend who had Leukaemia. Both of us seeking cures. Without going into too much detail, we arrived at what seemed an authentic Ayurvedic Clinic and they set to work. For forty-four consecutive days I received a variety of treatments, some of which were bizarre. I attended twice daily and received treatment from using the ancient form of Ayurveda, which is based on the 'Guru' system, and from a modern-trained Ayurvedic Doctor, trained in an updated version of Ayurveda, designed to meet western pharmaceutical demands. The cost for both was remarkably cheap.

Following that, I spent a further month in a Keralan 'Nature Cure' Centre, in the middle of a jungle. Watching elephants logging added to the sense of authenticity. In both systems, only safe, natural methods were used, with not a bleeping, radiating machine in sight. To me the idea you can not only treat but cure patients, without technology, was something novel. The end result of all this attention was my Arthritis symptoms disappeared. My circulation was restored. My normally-cold hands and feet felt as warm as toast. My rock-hard muscles were soft and relaxed and all the tension in my body was gone.

After several months in India, I left, inspired by what I had seen. I shall always be grateful to the humble, pot-bellied, Hindu 'Vaidya' (traditional Ayurvedic

Doctor), constantly standing on one leg, muttering mantras and counting his Mala beads, who tended to me. This curious man, who spoke no English, did more for me in a month with his massage and herbs than any 'scientific' Doctor ever did with their drugs. I had met my first authentic natural healer. What also struck me about him, wasn't just the Religious and Cultural strangeness of the man, which at first sight would cause most westerners to dismiss him, but the extent of his knowledge. I was shown a library of remedies, written on Papyrus, hundreds of years old, passed down from generation to generation within his family. Ancient wisdom, stemming from generations of trial and error. So impressed was I, I went on to study Ayurveda, 'Nature Cure' and other natural healing methods.

My discovery of natural healing was incredibly good news. So much so I excitedly tried to share my new-found knowledge with my Western-trained Doctor. I will never forget his disdainful dismissal. I did not know then but I have learned since, this closed-minded affliction, endemic amongst pharmaceutically-trained, western Doctors, is called 'Doctor Brain'.

Stress

We live in a highly stressful world. The effect on our nervous systems and psyche, from prolonged stress, is significant and cumulative. Tens of millions lack peace of mind, triggering a cascade of physical disorders and addictions. Those who aren't self-tranquillizing are on a cocktail of harmful psychiatric drugs.

Thoughts and emotions can powerfully affect brain, endocrine and immune system function. When we are stressed, specific hormones are secreted which allow us to run faster or fight harder. However, if sustained for longer periods of time, they inhibit the immune system. Chronic stress can trigger physical and psychological disorders and exacerbate existing ones. In a 2010 study, researchers in the Netherlands proved high levels of cortisol, a stress hormone, damage the cardiovascular system.

What other disorders does stress cause or influence? Almost anything you can think of. Asthma, Diabetes, Obesity, depression and anxiety, heartburn, IBS, Arthritis, accelerated aging and premature death. Stress produces tension in both mind and body via the 'Fight or Flight' response. We become angry or fearful. Our breathing becomes shallow, our thinking feels like wading through treacle. Try learning something new when your mind is 'foggy', concentration poor and memory non-existent. Cortisol blocks the creation of new synapses in the brain, preventing learning. Under stress, making even simple choices can initiate a crisis. Prolonged tension leads to high blood pressure, restricted blood, lymph and nerve flow, and impaired digestion. Tension also influences our acid/alkali balance. If you test the ph of your saliva when under stress, you find it is acidic.

Dis-stress creates uncomfortable thoughts and feelings, so we adopt ways to distract us. Turning up the volume on the radio, reaching for alcohol, food, sex, gambling and drugs. We 'self-harm' because all of these activities, while providing distraction (we lose ourselves in them temporarily), have negative consequences. Alcoholism, obesity, sex addiction, financial loss and drug addiction. Physical and psychological disorders may arise, or existing conditions worsen.

"Worry and stress affect the circulation, the heart, the glands, the whole nervous system, and profoundly affects heart action"

Charles W. Mayo, M.D

STRESS CURVE

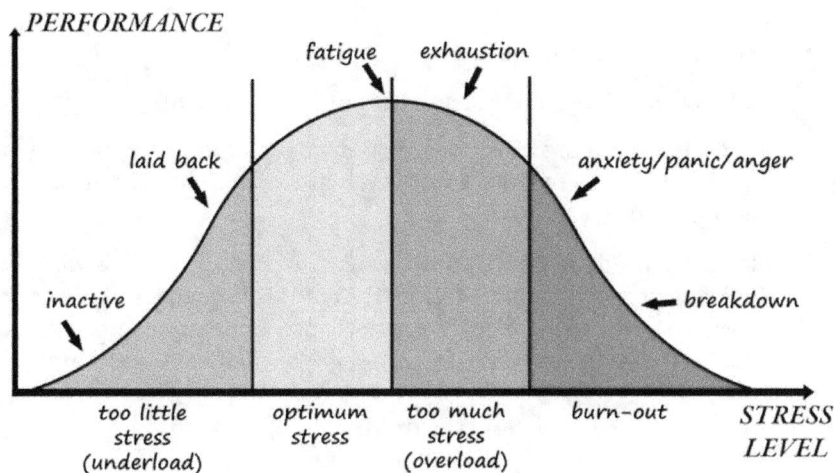

The Stress Curve chart above highlights the relationship between stress and performance. You can see that some stress is good for you. Too much, however, is bad.

There are four distinct phases of stress.

Too little stress

Optimum stress

Overload

Burn-out

As stress starts to rise, performance improves, until you reach optimum stress and peak performance. To perform well, we aim to stay in the 'optimum performance' phase. Unfortunately most of us are experiencing high stress levels and entering the later phases: fatigue, exhaustion, ill-health, breakdown and burnout.

Which phase are you in?

What Do We Know About Stress?

- Its effects are cumulative.

- Most of us are unaware of how tense we are. We are not in touch with our bodies and do not know ourselves.

- If a stressful situation is not resolved, eventually we will be forced to resolve it.

- A minor event can tip people over the edge.

- Burying one's head in the sand does not make problems go away.

- If you think you are 'mad' or 'going mad', you are not. Your body and mind are reacting to stress exactly as they should. You need EDUCATION more than medication.

- Relationships do not break down when life is good and all is well. They break down when severely tested. If a marriage or relationship does not have a strong foundation, it can collapse under pressure. Are your relationship's foundations strong enough to weather life's storms?

Sources of Stress

Physical

Illness. The adrenal glands are operating constantly trying to cope with inflammatory, nerve and other disorders. Bacteria, viruses, fungi and parasites drain the body's resources. Congestion and stagnation of blood, lymph, skin, liver, kidneys, nerve channels and bowel lead to the accumulation of toxins and metabolic wastes. Constipation and lack of physical activity are major contributors. Eating meat and poor food combinations causes putrefaction and auto-intoxication. Poisoning your body with your own wastes.

Chemical and heavy metal poisoning via food, air, water, vaccines and pharmaceutical drugs.

Energetic imbalances: electrical cables, cell phone transmitters, computers, mobile phones.

Radiation from irradiated food, medical devices, airport scanners and x-rays, nuclear power plants and depleted uranium, used in munitions.

Psychological

Toxic emotions and thoughts. Fear, anxiety, anger and frustration lead to physical and psychological tension. These can include 'spiritual' blockages, where you are divorced from your true 'Self'.

Discord between your inner and outer world is a major cause of stress. When your inner desires conflict with your outer experience. When you try to live the life that is expected of you, rather than the life your spirit craves.

Relationships, with mankind divided and set against each other. Divorce, Feminism, homosexuality, political correctness, attacks on Religion. Schools are 'dumbed down'. Politics is a 'circus' dominated by professional liars. The media swamp us with sensation, propaganda, 'dark' programming, constant fear, base language, and immorality. These draw us away from our true 'Sattvic' nature. (Sattvic, in Ayurveda, means having a serene, harmonious, balanced mind or attitude)

Poverty is a major cause of stress and illness. Poor quality housing, inner city violence and crime, financial insecurity, unemployment, homelessness, drugs.

Nutritional Deficiency

I previously mentioned **Nutritional Neuroscience** with regard to psychological stress. This is the effect of a lack of vital nutrients on psychological health, such as the 'B' (stress) vitamins, which are manufactured in the gut. What kinds of conditions upset our minds and emotions? There are a few.

- Medical conditions such as Crohn's disease, ulcerative colitis, Celiac Disease or persistent diarrhoea.

- Eating disorders, like anorexia or bulimia.

- Medicines disrupt the body's ability to absorb and break down nutrients. They also slow the transit time of waste products out of the body.

- Self-neglect. Failing to take proper care of oneself. e.g. Drug addicts and alcoholics.

- Eating nutrient-poor junk and industrial food.

- Physical disability, or other impairment, can make it difficult for you to cook and shop for food. Limited knowledge of how to preserve nutrients during cooking.

- Eating an incorrect diet for your Constitutional Type ('One man's meat is another man's poison')

- Undereating. Common in the elderly.

Millions are overweight, yet malnourished, from eating 'empty' calories. In Asia, where food is an important part of the social fabric, they are catching up fast with obesity and disease. 1 billion people around the world are today classed as clinically obese. In the UK, the most common causes of malnutrition in children are long-term health conditions which either cause low appetite, disrupt the normal process of digestion, or cause the body to have an increased demand for energy. Examples include childhood cancers, congenital heart disease, cystic fibrosis and cerebral palsy.

"Where on Earth Do I Start?!"

It is very easy to look at all the above and feel overwhelmed. I felt the same when I looked at my own unhappy life. We live in a very toxic world, with many stressors. The solution for me was to go back to nature, to return to simplicity, to embrace that powerful, yet suppressed, desire for freedom that was always a fundamental part of me. I did not want to 'DO'. I needed to 'BE'. Recognition of this is not 'cowardice'. Since when is living in accordance with your true nature cowardly? It is freedom. When the elderly are dying and asked 'What regrets do you have in life?' they all say the same. 'I wish I had really lived'. That isn't to say that duty and responsibility do not have their place but if you are weighed down, unhappy, depressed, suicidal, in what way is this beneficial to those around you? Are they so selfish they would contain you, imprison you in a life that is causing you suffering? If they truly love you, they would want the best for you. Ownership is not love.

If you feel overwhelmed, ask yourself the question I posed many pages ago. "Do you want to live or do you want to die?" If you want to live, you will look at all your sources of stress and resolve them. Make a list and then prioritize it. Take the top 5 stressors and resolve them. Then the next 5. Ask yourself, "What do I need to do to change this?" Switch off the TV and the smartphone, get rid of distractions and make being happy your most important project. Take it one step at a time. Do not feel overwhelmed. Be strong and have courage. You can repair relationships, become more loving, strip out all the junk and unnecessary rubbish that is clogging up your body, soul and mind. Be determined, stay focussed, approach it lightly, in a positive frame of mind and it will happen. Call it your **'Happiness Project'**.

Controlling a Troubled Mind

As you can see, the list of stressors is varied and lengthy, involving dietary, environmental and social factors. The idea you can eat some Goji berries or drink Noni Juice and your health will immediately improve is unlikely. If you wish to be healthy and happy, you need to look at every aspect of your lives. Manage your stress and control what you are feeding body and mind.

Where you are unable to change something, like your environment, all is not lost. One of the most iconic symbols in Asia is the Lotus Flower, which grows in muddy water, yet produces wonderful blossoms. We, too, can thrive despite adverse circumstances.

When balanced, our minds are calm, clear-thinking and a useful tool. When out of balance they become tyrannical. Fearful thoughts, angry thoughts, useless thoughts, sexual thoughts, dark and repetitive thoughts. Constantly swirling around in our mental soup. We feel powerless to settle the mind because we have been trained to look outward for solutions, never inward. We do not believe we can control or change our thoughts. Most of the time, we are not even aware of what we are thinking.

On both Online Health Coaching programs and retreats we teach you how to observe, then change your thinking so that, like the Lotus flower, you can blossom in a challenging environment. Most people operate on automatic-pilot, in a kind of trance-like state. Eating, walking, driving, talking, with little awareness of what they are thinking. The mind dwelling on the past or worrying about the future. Increasingly, we are glued to smartphones.

Just like computers, we have an input and an output. What we output reflects what has been input. We can program, or allow others to program, our minds with all kinds of beliefs and ideas. When we sit, unconsciously snacking, in front of a TV or movie screen, there is very little filtering of what we allow into our minds. As mentioned, previously, we are constantly told what to think, what to believe, what to eat, what to wear, who to like, who to hate, who is in and who is out. Passive acceptance of these messages is dangerous to our psychological health because much of what we see is scripted to deceive. To create a false view of reality. To re-write history, turn 'good' into 'bad' and 'bad' into 'good'. Medical dramas enthral us with gripping storylines while planting false ideas which we unthinkingly absorb.

The mind needs to be nourished with positive, powerful, loving, messages. Not hate, sensationalism, division, propaganda, immorality and 200 channels of stupefying rubbish. 'Garbage in, Garbage out'. Not only does media brainwashing shape our beliefs, it over-stimulates the nervous system. The rapidly changing images and roller-coaster ride of fear, excitement and anger, exhausts our adrenals and destroys our concentration until we end up unable to relax and addicted to the next stimuli. Eventually we become bored, needing ever-increasing sensation to capture and hold our attention.

A good place, therefore, to start reducing stress, is with the media. I am far happier today, not reading newspapers, watching TV, Hollywood movies or music videos. These mediums are dragging mankind into a very dark place.

The internet can do the same. Only you are able to actively select what you put into your mind, rather than passively accept what someone else wants to feed you. The internet provides alternative viewpoints the mainstream media will not present. Although that is rapidly changing as a handful of internet companies dominate. Alternative viewpoints are side-lined, un-indexed by search engines, or taken down.

Take care with your internet use. There is a price to be paid for over-doing it. The repetitive 'clack-clack-clackety-clack' of fingers on keyboards, irritates our nervous system. Addiction, electro-magnetic radiation, lack of exercise, eyestrain and poor posture also create stress. When our eyes are constantly switching between images we develop grasshopper minds.

If your mind is filled to overflowing or thinking feels like you are ploughing through a muddy field, follow the advice of Air Force fighter pilots. They have three steps to staying focussed.

1. Checklists. Write down what you need to know.

2. Cross-checking. If you have a long list of tasks, take the top 5 most important tasks and double-check they are completed.

3. Find mutual support. Have a friend, work colleague, buddy or family member who will back you up and spot anything you may miss.

What Have You Learned?

Well. Here we are at the end of our journey together. There is a lot to digest, so here's a recap. My aim in writing was to:

- Explain why we are sick and where disease is coming from.

- Guide you toward better health.

- Shed light on why Mainstream Medicine is unable to cure chronic disease.

- Point out the fallacy of managing disease, rather than healing it.

- Question whether those who claim authority over your body are working in your interests or their own?

- Explain why Alternative Medicine fails to cure, unless you have the right tools in your healing toolbox and know how to use them.

- Stress the critical importance of proper detoxification and elimination.

- Have you understand that, no matter how low you feel, or how desperate your situation, there is always hope. Never let any self-proclaimed expert or authority-figure take that away from you.

- Point out official experts and official studies are often wrong or misleading. Trust your own instincts.

- Educate you in how to heal yourself, rather than rely on those who do not really have an answer and do not know you.

- Have you focus on the right way to reverse disease and not waste time, energy and money on the wrong.

- Encourage you to reclaim power over what you are putting into your mouth and have you ask yourself whether what you are eating and drinking is building health or building disease? The apple or the doughnut.

- Inspire you to free yourself from addiction, using tools like juice-fasting, the 'Bitter' taste, EFT and 'Breaking the Chains' and dissolve the toxic emotions which drive you to self-tranquillize.

- Show you healing is not complicated. We just make it that way.

- Have you understand, at a deeper level, you are a wonderful creation, whose body is a Temple. That, no matter how poor your external environment, you can be the Lotus Flower.

- Encourage you to stick with ONE program and not be a grasshopper, bouncing from therapy to therapy. Just ensure it is the right program!

- Have you understand what 'over-medicalization' means and make you question whether you really need all those tests and procedures.

- Help you understand you are not healing a specific disorder or relieving a symptom but strengthening the body and giving it everything it needs to heal, so ALL your disorders will resolve.

- Have you understand healing is not dependent on diagnosis.

- Introduce you to forgotten healing knowledge.

- Remind you there are Laws of Nature which always bring consequences when violated.

- Remind you that, while violating Nature's Laws can cause disease, living in accordance with them can prevent and reverse it.

- Have you take action NOW and not wait and wait until your disease is so far gone it becomes more difficult to resolve, or you are dead.

- Point out that, without good health, material wealth is of little comfort. Your health is your greatest possession. Invest in it.

- Put you in touch with your inner SELF. To unite the outer part of you with the glorious, eternal inner you, neglected for so long.

- Let you know you do not need to do this alone. That support is available if you need it. To 'Seek and ye shall find'.

- Remind you of the positive qualities. That love is a vital ingredient in this fallen world. Without it, we are fearful, alone and empty. Love yourself. Respect yourself. Believe in yourself and have courage.

- Teach you that resistance in the mind causes resistance in the body. Learn forgiveness. Let go. Whatever is in the past, leave it in the past. Look forward, not backward.

- Inspire you, no matter your religion or beliefs, to dust off your soul, your spirit, the inner you, and shine brightly.

- Encourage you to take responsibility for your health and eliminate everything in your life that is an impediment to healing.

- Not stick with failure. If your Doctor is unwilling or unable to cure you, FIRE YOUR DOCTOR and CURE YOURSELF.

The Next Step

I have done my bit. Now it is your turn. To put into action what you have learned. To resist moving on to the next book, guru, telegenic TV Doctor or well-meaning friend, telling you they have a better, easier way. Or, if you do, at least you will do so with greater knowledge and understanding.

Remember why you are doing this...

"We all deserve a life of glowing health and vitality, free from pain and sickness, whether in Body, Mind or Spirit. It is our birthright. To be happy. To be at peace. To enjoy a long, healthy existence on this beautiful planet. To love ourselves, our families and our fellow man. To pass away peacefully in our sleep".

Worth striving for, don't you think? Take heart. We are in an Age of transition, where the planet will detox and mankind will have its own parasite-cleanse, before entering a brilliant New Age. Do not stay unhappy or unhealthy a day longer. Make a vow right now:

"**Today, I make this promise to myself. I am going to restore my health. Nothing is going to stand in my way. I am a unique and beautiful child of God (or Nature). No longer will I allow those who care nothing for me to destroy my health. I am taking back control of my life and when I experience moments of weakness, will not break. Instead I will use those moments to strengthen my resolve.**"

Well done. Now just do it. And when you have done it, let me know via the website, Facebook or email, how you fared. If you feel you are struggling or cannot do it alone, by all means get in touch.

Wishing you peace, happiness and the very best of health!

Paul Keenan

Appendix

What are Doshas?

The Doshas are a set of characteristics in India's Ayurvedic medicine, similar to the ancient Greek concept of "humours," which were unfortunately misused (and hence given a bad press) in the West. The three doshas: Vata (Air), Pitta (Fire) and Kapha (Earth or Water) are used to describe people based on their physical, mental, emotional and psychological characteristics. Each dosha reflects one or more of the base elements. Earth, Air, Fire and Water.

The Meaning of a "Dosha"

Ayurvedic traditions recognize and honour the uniqueness of each individual, but the highest virtue is balance. It is believed every person requires different ingredients for optimal health, to balance their doshas and their particular constitutional type. Ayurveda means "The Science (or Knowledge) of Life," while Dosha means each of three energies believed to circulate in the body and govern physiological activity. Every person possesses some of the qualities of all three doshas. The unique balance between Air, Fire, Earth & Water (Vata, Pitta, Kapha) determines a person's constitution, body type, and mental and emotional strengths and weaknesses.

Finding Your Dosha Type

Most people will have one predominant dosha, but others have two or all three in equal balance. Dozens of tests and resources are available online to help identify your Dosha.

The Three Doshas

Vata (Air)

Vata dosha is composed of the elements of air and space (or ether). Vata is dry, cool, light, clear and active. It governs breathing, elimination, motor skills and the senses.

People who have a Vata constitution are noticeably tall or short, with a light frame, small musculature, and low body fat. They usually have dry hair and skin, low body temperature and blood pressure, a small mouth and grey, brown or blue eyes.

Vata temperament is quick and clever, but impatient and lacking in stamina. Vata people are commonly active and creative, but they tend to sleep lightly and may be shy, anxious and insecure.

Vata imbalance can cause worries, insomnia, fluctuating appetite, cramps and constipation. Vata governs the other two doshas and is usually the first cause of illness or disease. Foods that are warm, moist, mildly spicy and well-cooked, balance and contain Vata.

Pitta (Fire)

Pitta is predominantly fire with some water. It is hot, light, liquid, sour, sharp and oily. Pitta governs metabolism and digestive processes of the mind, body and spirit; intelligence and understanding; hunger and thirst; and the fiery emotions of anger, hate and jealousy.

Pitta people are of medium build, with fair skin that may show freckles or blemishes, a medium-sized mouth, and blue or hazel eyes.

Those with pitta temperament are organized, ambitious and driven but easily irritated. They love knowledge and possess leadership abilities. Although they are competitive, controlling and judgmental, they usually accomplish a great deal. They have strong digestive systems, moderate stamina and enjoy physical activity.

Pitta governs the small intestine, stomach, skin, eyes, fat, sweat and blood. Imbalance often shows as impatience, hostility, and emotional outbursts which can affect these physical areas.

Pitta should avoid cigarettes and anything heating or aggravating to the body's systems. Foods to soothe pitta are cool, sweet, bitter and astringent.

Kapha (Earth/Water)

Kapha combines the elements of 'Water' and 'Earth', and has the most physicality of the three doshas. Kapha is cool, heavy, dense, slow, and liquid, and governs the joints, strength, the heart, lungs and wound healing.

Kapha people are usually heavier than other types due to slower metabolism, with cool or oily skin, dark eyes, large lips and thick, wavy hair. They are relaxed, patient, compassionate, and steady. They neither learn nor accept change easily, but they have steady energy and stamina. They may seem withdrawn or impassionate.

Excess Kapha results in emotional attachment and clinginess, greed, and envy. It can also contribute to weight gain, lethargy, congestion and allergies.

Foods with the opposite properties to earth and water, (i.e. cold, heavy and mucus-forming) are warm, light, dry, spicy and bitter and will balance kapha. These types do well on vegan and vegetarian diets.

Chakras

The Sanskrit word 'Chakra' literally translates to wheel or disk. In yoga, meditation, and Ayurveda, this term refers to wheels of energy throughout the body. Chakras are energy centres running from the top of the head to the base of the spine. There are 7 chakras, which have important influences on the body and mind. I will not go into detail since there are more than enough concepts and techniques in the book for you to absorb and utilize.

Learning More

To learn more about Ayurveda, I recommend books by either David Frawley or Vasant Lad.

May I Ask a Favour?

Did you enjoy the book? If you think it is helpful and deserves to be brought to the attention of a wider audience, you can help.

WRITE A POSITIVE BOOK REVIEW (wherever you purchased it).

If you know someone who is sick, depressed or might benefit, send them a link to the book, website, or buy them a copy.

If you use social media, 'Like', 'Share', 'Follow', tag, discuss, recommend, bookmark, link, forward, chat, message, tweet, carrier pigeon and whatever else you feel will bring the book to peoples' notice. Many are suffering who don't need to. Help spread the word!

Create A Family!

Do not let this be the end of our journey together. Another step in the Bypass Age revolution is to create an online community. On our ToDo list is setting up a member area on the website. Members are entitled to special deals like discounts on coaching and retreats. Also check the **Special Offers** page. Keep up with our health and wellness blog and sign up to our Newsletter. I promise not to overwhelm you with nagging emails! If the member area is not yet set up, bookmark the blog so you can keep track of new developments.

If you are in Thailand, come and pitch in on a retreat. We are always glad of assistance, preparing food or making juices. If you are a raw foodie, we would love to see what you can conjure up!

Retreats and Online Health Coaching

As you have gathered from these pages, I oversee **Health & Wellness Retreats** in Thailand. If you find following a healing program at home a challenge, a retreat may be just what you need. Many guests sign up for the expertise and support we provide and to kick-start their healing or wellness efforts. Our focus at Antarana is on providing individual programs but group retreats are growing. The Homestay is particularly popular.

My goal in establishing a retreat and writing this book was to honour my mother and create a lasting legacy. The completion of 'Fire Your Doctor Cure Yourself' and creation of Antarana Health & Wellness is the fulfilment of that dream. Our small holistic 'family' share the same natural healing vision. We are caring and extremely dedicated to helping others. Adhering, at all times, to the philosophy I encountered in Kerala, India, "A Guest is a God"

The foundation of our cleansing (detox) and healing programs is juice-fasting. Using fresh, organic, seasonal fruits and vegetables. This is because we agree with the ancient's view. You must stop eating until your body is cleansed and you are well. Our juice-fasting programs are surprisingly easy. They are also effective. That is why 50% of our customers come back again and again. I should point out we are not a high-class luxury spa, nor a Swiss clinic, operating like clockwork, with Doctors in white coats and stethoscopes and nurses in crisp, starched uniforms. Nor are we an insect-plagued hut on the beach or a retreat 'mill' with Spartan accommodation. We try to strike a balance between quality accommodation, personal attention and serious programs. We even build in fun days where you can go and be a tourist or flop on the beach for the day. Thailand has had some bad press but that's the media for you. If there was really any danger, we simply wouldn't live here. We have children, too. Some combine a holiday with wellness. If you want to go to the beach every day, or sight-see, we make up drinks to take with you.

Those unable to attend a retreat can benefit instead from **Online Health Coaching**. This is where we connect online and work together to resolve whatever your health or wellness issue is. With today's technology, connecting via Skype, Hangouts (or whichever you prefer) is easy. No matter where you are or what you are doing. It beats trudging down to the Doctor's surgery in rain or snow and leaving with a bag full of side effects. No worries about parking, fighting through traffic, or sitting in a busy waiting room. Our Online Appointment Scheduler allows you to choose the time and sends out automatic reminders to your phone or email. No more forgotten appointments! Cost of coaching may seem high but a 1 hour coaching session (which can be broken up), for you, can involve hours of investigation and preparation, for me. I don't use automated, generic programs. Programs are tailored just for you.

Where Does The Name Antarana Come from?

Antarana is the name of a Peruvian village surrounded by stunning mountains. Since every name I thought of had already been taken, it seemed as good as any.

A word about the various mentions of what I do and where, within the book. We live in a world where you need to be proactive in putting yourself, your products or your company in front of eyeballs. If you do not, you will simply not be seen. The following is a list of programs we currently offer. You can check in on the Retreats page on the website every now and again to see what's new. If you don't see the program you want, email, or use the free chat, and ask us to design a program for you. If you decide to come, we would love to see you!

PROGRAMS AT ANTARANA

DETOX RETREATS

Super Juice!

Master Cleanse

Fluoride Detox

Heavy Metal Detox

WELLNESS RETREATS

Reverse Diabetes

Life After Cancer

Incurables

ONLINE HEALTH COACHING

Life After Cancer

Reverse Diabetes

Incurables At Home

Fluoride Detox

Heavy Metal Detox

Book a session via the website or email:

www.antarana.com/online-coaching

healthcoach@antarana.com

Contact Us

Information: info@antarana.com

Customer Service: customerservice@antarana.com

Health Coach: healthcoach@antarana.com

Retreat Manager: retreats@antarana.com

Special Offers: offers@antarana.com

Website: www.antarana.com

Giving Back

I very much believe in the importance of helping others. The following deserving causes will receive a percentage from book sales. Details on the Website's 'Giving Back' page.

'Power of Love' Children's Home

Rescue Paws, a dog charity

'Lem', a Thai villager with Stage IV Lung Cancer

ABOUT THE AUTHOR

Paul Keenan has lived at least 3 lifetimes. Three marriages, three children, three wars, three careers, and three powerful motorcycles, wiped out, when racing. Paul has windsurfed in three different oceans and 'pitched his tent' in over 50 countries. An engineer in the British Royal Navy; market-trader, selling second-hand, brand-name sweaters in gypsy markets in the Algarve ("for fun!"), Paul spent 6 years as an I.T. manager for a cosmetics company... a highlight of which was winning a UK-wide technology award... before going on to run his own computer business until, as he puts it, his 'brains blew up'. After a 20-yr struggle with poor health, in the last decade Paul has found purpose and fulfilment running a Health and Wellness Retreat in a beach resort in Thailand. It is easy to understand why Paul knows so much about meditation and mindfulness. He needed it!

Feeling the need to increase awareness of the failings of modern medicine, and how natural healing offers solutions, Paul decided to take time out from running detox, healing retreats and online health coaching, to write 'Fire Your Doctor Cure Yourself.'

To learn more about Paul, Visit www.antarana.com

Follow him on Facebook www.facebook.com/PaulKeenanAuthor/

Paul also blogs at www.antarana.com/blog

COMING NEXT

FIRE YOUR PSYCHIATRIST

by

Paul Keenan

The French were very good at separating the head from the body, with their Guillotine. Unsurprisingly, people did not find it a healing experience. So why does Psychiatry separate the head from the body and expect people to improve?

In a world where drugging of the masses has become normal, Paul Keenan uses straightforward language to demolish the Psychiatric nonsense being peddled by so-called mental health experts. 6 million children in the U.S. are being given Class II narcotics for behaviour that can be corrected by better parenting, proper nutrition, cutting out 'excito-toxic' sugars, removing toxic heavy metals, and reducing poverty. Millions of adults are given 'chemical coshes' because they are suffering toxic STRESS, caused by toxic politicians, toxic medicine, toxic media, toxic food, toxic relationships and a toxic environment.

The consequences of swallowing poisonous fluoride compounds, otherwise known as 'anti-depressants', are addiction, suicide, impotence and permanent brain changes, for benefits which have been exaggerated. We truly are a Zombie Nation.

Natural and Alternatives remedies are unfairly vilified for a lack of scientific evidence to support them. Psychiatry has even less (has anyone ever seen a test for a chemical imbalance of the brain?) yet is fully supported by government. 25% of Americans are reported as having a mental disorder. One quarter of the population. Are these people really 'mad'?

To find out more or reserve your copy, email info@antarana.com